COMBATING EMERGING INFECTIOUS DISEASES

Using the Financial Action Task

FORCE NATIONAL RISK ASSESSMENT STRATEGY

In memoriam

DR. ANGELA
EITERHEBHE ESOIMEME
1956–2020

EHI ERIC ESOIMEME

DR. ANGELA EITERHEBHE ESOIMEME

E-FOUR & AAF
TRAINING AND CONSULTING FIRM

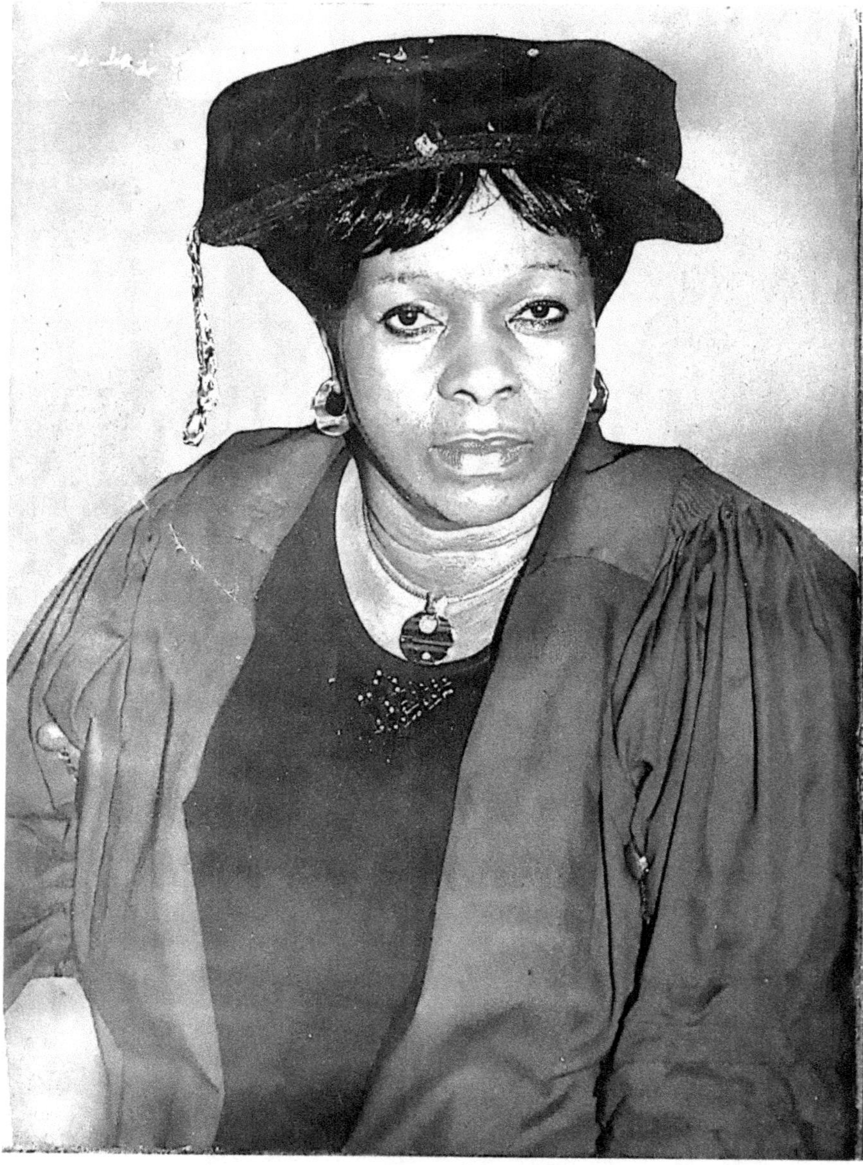

IN MEMORIAM

DR. ANGELA EITERHEBHE ESOIMEME

1956–2020

DISCLAIMER

The information contained in this book is intended for the purpose of general information and should not be used to substitute for the individual expertise and judgement of healthcare professionals.

ISBN-10: 978-2787-92-2

ISBN-13: 978-978-2787-92-7

Published by E-Four and AAF.

No. 2, Dapo Bode Thomas Street,

Off Thorburn Street, Via Montgomery/Commercial Avenue.

To my beloved mother and best friend, Dr. Angela Eiterhebhe Esoimeme for always being there for me and for assisting me in this project. I will always love you, Mama.

ACKNOWLEDGEMENTS

I take this opportunity to express my deep sense of gratitude to my mother, Dr. Angela Eiterhebhe Esoimeme for her encouragement and support throughout my life and for contributing valuable content to this excellent book.

I must also express my sincere gratitude to Mr. Ian Ross for his continuous bouts of encouragement and support and for contributing the foreword to this book. I am heartened by his absolute endorsement of this publication.

I am eternally grateful to God for our families and friends who stood by us over the years. I cannot thank you enough for your support and kindness and for your desire to keep my mother's legacy alive. I owe you a debt of gratitude.

TABLE OF CONTENTS

FOREWORD 10

PREFACE 12

ABOUT THE AUTHORS 17

I. EHI ERIC ESOIMEME 17

II. DR. ANGELA EITERHEBHE ESOIMEME 18

LIST OF ACRONYMS AND ABBREVIATIONS 20

GLOSSARY OF TERMINOLOGY 27

CHAPTER 1 INTRODUCTION TO EMERGING INFECTIOUS DISEASES: STEMMING THE TIDE 40

1.1. EMERGING INFECTIOUS DISEASES THAT HAVE BEEN IDENTIFIED IN THE PAST 40 YEARS 42

1.1.1. COVID-19 43

1.1.2. Middle East Respiratory Syndrome (MERS) 45

1.1.3. Severe Acute Respiratory Syndrome (SARS) 48

1.1.4. Ebola Virus Disease 50

1.1.5. Marburg Virus Disease 57

1.1.6. Avian and Other Zoonotic Influenza 59

1.1.7. Seasonal Influenza 63

1.1.8. Pandemic Influenza 71

1.1.9. Human Immunodeficiency Virus (HIV) 74

1.2. THE GLOBAL APPROACH TO COMBATING INFECTIOUS DISEASES 75

1.2.1. The World Health Organization 76

1.2.2. United States Centers for Disease Control and Prevention 80

1.2.3. United Kingdom's Department of Health 85

1.2.4. Nigeria Centre for Disease Control 91

CHAPTER 2 OVERVIEW OF THE METHODOLOGY TO ASSESS PUBLIC HEALTH RISKS AND EVENTS AT THE NATIONAL LEVEL 94
2.1. UNITED STATES 101
2.1.1.Identify Threats and Hazards of Concern 102
2.1.2.Give Threats and Hazards Context 104
2.1.3.Establish Capability Targets 104
2.2 UNITED KINGDOM 106
2.2.1. Identifying Risks 106
2.2.2. Assessing Risks 107
2.2.3 Comparison of the Risks 108
2.3 NIGERIA 109
2.3.1 Identifying Specific Disaster Risk(s) 110
2.3.2 Analysing the Disaster Risk(s) 110
2.3.3 Monitoring Disaster Risks 111
2.3.4 Evaluating Disaster Risk Assessed, Updating and Disseminating Information to All Stakeholders 111
CHAPTER 3 THE FINANCIAL ACTION TASK FORCE'S APPROACH TO NATIONAL RISK ASSESSMENT 113
3.1 NATIONAL RISK ASSESSMENT 115
3.2 STAGES OF MONEY LAUNDERING NATIONAL RISK ASSESSMENT 120
3.2.1 Identification 120
3.2.2 Analysis 123
3.2.3 Evaluation 125
CHAPTER 4 ASSESSING THE RISKS OF EMERGING INFECTIOUS DISEASES WITH THE FINANCIAL ACTION TASK FORCE RISK ASSESSMENT STRATEGY 130
4.1. FIRST STAGE: IDENTIFICATION 130
4.2.SECOND STAGE: ANALYSIS 134
4.3.THIRD STAGE: EVALUATION 137

CHAPTER 5 RISK CONTROL MEASURES 146

5.1 REDUCING THE SPREAD OF DISEASE: INFECTION CONTROL & RESPIRATORY AND HAND HYGIENE ... 147

5.2 INTERNATIONAL TRAVEL, BORDER RESTRICTIONS AND SCREENING 149

5.3 CLOSURE OF SCHOOLS AND RESTRICTIONS ON PUBLIC GATHERINGS AND PUBLIC TRANSPORT 152

5.4 FACEMASKS AND RESPIRATORS 154

5.5 CONTROLLING INFECTION IN HEALTH-CARE SETTINGS 155

5.5.1 Care for People with Suspected or Confirmed COVID-19 155

5.5.2 Care for People Who Recovered From COVID-19 163

5.6 CONTACT TRACING 165

5.6.1 Contact Identification 166

5.6.2 Contact Listing 167

5.6.3 Contact Follow-Up 169

5.7 TREATMENT 171

INDEX 172

EHI ERIC ESOIMEME'S PUBLICATIONS 183

FOREWORD

This book provides us with a striking reality of how an awful global event, such as COVID-19, imbues with global financial crime prevention. It is easy to overlook the scale of money laundering as a pandemic itself with so many contexts, nuances, and an array of recording processes and reporting channels of money laundering.

In fact, many would not see a pandemic of infectious disease and financial crime as entirely different topics. Hence, qualitative analysis to unearth these unquestionably linked issues was needed.

With this concept, Ehi Eric Esoimeme has produced a coruscating publication with skill, flair, and innovation that has become his trademark.

I cannot emphasise enough the value of this book as a working resource to keep the threats and implications of money laundering in yet another context at our conscious level. This book, with its clear rationale, makes the case for how applying a risk assessment strategy can make a major contribution to combating emerging infectious diseases.

Ian Ross

Director, Compliance & Training

Accredited Counter Fraud Specialist

"Listed expert" *Cour pénale* internationale (The International Court of Justice, The Hague)

Fellow: Chartered Management Institute

Trainer: Association of Certified Anti-Money Laundering Specialists

PREFACE

The coronavirus disease 2019 (COVID-19) outbreak highlights the ongoing threat to global health posed by emerging infectious diseases. As the crisis fades away, attention has turned towards the lessons to be learned for preparedness and response to emerging infectious diseases.

Before 2009, national pandemic response actions were guided by global risk assessment and pandemic phases. This changed after the experience of pandemic A(H1N1)2009. Countries have now been advised by the World Health Organization to base response actions on their own assessment of national pandemic risk and severity, and the corresponding national pandemic phase.

In national pandemic preparedness plans, the national pandemic phase is typically represented by a grading system to indicate the level of alert or seriousness. Changes in the severity of the national pandemic phase can be used in a scenario to communicate the level of pandemic "threat" and to prompt the corresponding response actions set out in the country's pandemic influenza preparedness plan.

PURPOSE OF THE BOOK

This research seeks to enhance the collective understanding of the national risk-assessment process for managing the risk(s) of new and emerging infections arising anywhere in the world and draws upon principles set out under Recommendation 1 of the Financial Action Task Force's International Standards on Combating Money Laundering and the Financing of Terrorism and Proliferation 2012 (updated 2019). Recommendation 1 of the Financial Action Task Force Standards requires, amongst others, that countries identify, analyse, and evaluate their money laundering and terrorist financing risks and apply anti-money laundering and combating the financing of terrorism measures that are commensurate with the identified risks.

TARGET AUDIENCE

The concepts in this book are aimed at state agencies, such as emergency management, partner organizations, other jurisdictional public health agencies, health care coalitions, community-based partners, and other jurisdictional stakeholders.

CONTENT OF THE BOOK

The first chapter of this book examines the subject of emerging infectious diseases in relation to their definition, history, symptoms, transmission, incubation period, diagnosis, treatment, and prevention and expounds on the response planning strategies that have been developed by the World Health Organization, the United States of America, the United Kingdom, and Nigeria to attempt to identify new infectious threats as they emerge to facilitate a timely response, including control.

Chapter 2 analyses the process for conducting a risk assessment at the national level with a focus on the national risk assessment strategy of the United States of America, the United Kingdom and Nigeria.

Chapter 3 analyses the process for conducting a risk assessment at the national level with a focus on the national risk assessment strategy of the Financial Action Task Force.

Chapter 4 gives an explicit explanation for how countries can identify, analyse, and evaluate emerging and potential infectious threats to public health both nationally and internationally using the Financial Action Task Force risk-assessment strategy with a focus on COVID-19.

Chapter 5 expounds on the measures that can help curb the spread of infectious diseases with a primary focus on COVID-19.

Design/Methodology/Approach

The terminology and methodology of this research are based on the guidance of the Financial Action Task Force, which presents a process for conducting a risk assessment at the national level. Risk in the context of money laundering and terrorist financing is a function of three factors: (1) threat, (2) vulnerability, (3) and consequence. The money laundering and terrorist financing risk assessment involve making judgements about these three factors. This book followed the three key stages identified in the Financial Action Task Force guidance of (1) identification, (2) analysis, and (3) evaluation.

FINDINGS

The research determined that countries can use the Financial Action Task Force risk assessment strategy to identify, analyse, and evaluate emerging and potential infectious threats to public health, both nationally and internationally, and take action, including officially shutting the country's airports, seaports, and borders, while still developing medical countermeasures, such as vaccines and treatments, and apply resources aimed at ensuring that risks are mitigated effectively. This includes early identification and systematic rapid isolation of cases under appropriate Infection Prevention and Control (IPC) measures, timely and comprehensive contact tracing, disinfection of infectious materials, and appropriate use of personal protective equipment.

Isolation of infected patients with appropriate IPC measures has been shown to effectively stop the spread of disease in previous outbreaks. Good outbreak control relies on a good laboratory service, safe burials, and social mobilization. Community engagement is key to successfully controlling outbreaks. Raising awareness of risk factors for COVID-19 infection and protective measures (including vaccination) that individuals can take is an effective way to reduce human transmission.

Originality/Value

Although the literature on risk assessment is extensive, there is little that is specific to the assessment of emerging public health threats at the national level. This research provides further explanation of the risk assessment process for identifying, understanding, and reducing emerging and potential infectious threats to public health both nationally and internationally with the Financial Action Task Force risk assessment methodology. This is the only research to adopt this kind of approach.

ABOUT THE AUTHORS

I. EHI ERIC ESOIMEME

Ehi Eric Esoimeme is the managing partner of *E-Four and AAF* (a global consultancy firm that also offers training and education to financial institutions on anti-money laundering compliance). His area of specialism and expertise is in countering financial crime. This is categorized into regulatory law, substantive law, and professional compliance guidance in terms of strategic management of money laundering risks and vulnerabilities. Ehi has now used his experience in the area of risk assessment and mitigation to write this book.

Ehi's skill and knowledge in the field of the financial crime space are drawn from his many years of experience as a researcher in anti-money laundering laws and policies, counter-fraud measures, and anti-corruption strategies. So far, Ehi has authored more than 30 publications, including seven books on money laundering law/banking law. Ehi's second book titled *The Risk-Based Approach to Combating Money Laundering and Terrorist Financing* became a bestseller on Amazon for banking law. Ehi's sixth book titled *The Risk-Based Approach to Combating Modern Slavery* has received many commendations from both academic researchers and anti-money laundering professionals.

Ehi received a bachelor's degree in law from the University of Lagos and holds a master's degree in international banking law and anti-money laundering compliance from Cardiff University.

Ehi is a fellow of the Institute of Management Consultants and a senior member of the Risk Management Association of Nigeria. Ehi currently sits on the editorial board of the *International Journal of Law and Society* and reviews manuscripts for several international journals.

Ehi has served as the deputy editor in chief of DSC Publications Ltd., a leader and pioneer in legal publishing in Nigeria. As deputy editor in chief, Ehi successfully completed two major projects for the firm. The first was published in 13 volumes, while the second was published in seven volumes.

II. DR. ANGELA EITERHEBHE ESOIMEME

Dr. Angela Eiterhebhe Esoimeme (née Eitokpah) is the mother of Ehi Eric Esoimeme Esq. Dr. Esoimeme was born on November 1, 1956, in Vom, Plateau State. She attended the prestigious Queens College, Yaba, Lagos, where she was awarded the Federal Government Scholarship for Academic Excellence and the Shell B.P. Scholarship for Academic Excellence because of her academic brilliance. At Queen's College, she won annual prizes for academic excellence. Then she proceeded to the prestigious College of Medicine at the University of Lagos where she obtained a bachelor of medicine, bachelor of surgery degree and was awarded the Federal Government Scholarship for Academic Excellence. Dr. Esoimeme also obtained a master's in public health at the College of Medicine at the University of Lagos and a certificate in human resources management.

Dr. Esoimeme started her medical career as a house officer at the Lagos University Teaching Hospital, Idi-Araba, in 1980 and was later promoted to the position of chief medical officer in 1999 at the Staff Clinic, Lagos University Teaching Hospital, Idi-Araba. Dr. Angela Esoimeme reached the pinnacle of her career as head of the Department of Family Medicine, Lagos University Teaching Hospital, Idi-Araba, Surulere, Lagos, for 14 years, until she retired from her work as a consultant and family physician.

Dr. Esoimeme was a fellow of the West African College of Physicians and a member of the Society of Family Physicians of Nigeria, Medical and Dental Consultants in Nigeria, West African College of Physicians, National Postgraduate Medical College of Nigeria, Nigerian Medical Association, Health and Environmental Rights, Medical Women's Association of Nigeria, World Organization of Family Doctors, and Lagos University Medical Society. She was the secretary of the Medical Women's Association of Nigeria, Lagos state branch from 1999 to 2001. Her legacy includes training more than 60 doctors over the course of her career.

She will forever be missed.

LIST OF ACRONYMS AND ABBREVIATIONS

AAR: After action review

ABHR: Alcohol-based hand rub

AFB: Acid fast bacilli

AFP: Acute Flaccid Paralysis

AFRO: Regional Office for Africa (at WHO)

ALT: Alanine aminotransferase

AML/CFT: Anti-Money Laundering / Countering the Financing of Terrorism

AMR: Antimicrobial Resistance

AST: Aspartate aminotransferase

BSL: Biosafety level

CBC: Complete blood count

CCHFV: Crimean-Congo haemorrhagic fever virus

CDC: Centers for Disease Control and Prevention (the United States of America)

COMBI: Communication for Behavioural Impact

CSF: Cerebrospinal fluid

CSO: Civil Society Organizations

CT: cycle threshold

CTU: Covid-19 Treatment Unit

DNFBPs: Designated Non-Financial Businesses and Professions

DRC: Democratic Republic of Congo

DSMB: Data and Safety Monitoring Board

EBOV: Ebola virus

EC: European Commission

ECDC: European Center for Disease Prevention and Control

EMRO: WHO Regional Office for the Eastern Mediterranean

EOC: Emergency Operations Centre

ERCC: Emergency Response Coordination Centre

ETC: Ebola treatment centre

EtD: evidence-to-decision

ETU: Ebola treatment unit

EURO: WHO Regional Office for Europe

EVD: Ebola virus disease (acute EVD refers to laboratory-confirmed (positive viremia) and symptomatic Ebola virus disease)

EWRS: Early Warning and Response System

FATF: Financial Action Task Force

FEC: Federal Executive Council

FIU: Financial Intelligence Units

Gavi: The Vaccine Alliance

GCP: good clinical practice

GDG: Guideline Development Group

GERD: Gastro-oesophageal reflux disease

GNI: Gross National Income

GPEI: Global Polio Eradication Initiative

GRADE: Grading of Recommendations Assessment, Development and Evaluation

GRC: Guideline Review Committee

GSC: Guideline Steering Committee

HCID: High-Consequence Infectious Disease

HCW: Healthcare worker

HEPA: High-efficiency particulate air filter

HFRS: Haemorrhagic fever with renal syndrome

HQ: headquarters

HSC: Health Security Committee

IEC: Information, Education and Communication

IHR (2005): International Health Regulations (2005)

IHR MEF: International Health Regulations (2005) Monitoring and Evaluation Framework

IHR NFP: International Health Regulations National Focal Point

INFOSAN FP: International Food Safety Authorities Network Focal Point

IPC: Infection Prevention and Control

ITSON: Integrated Training for Surveillance Officers in Nigeria

JEE: Joint External Evaluation

LFT: Liver function test

LGA: Local Government Area

LHF: Lassa haemorrhagic fever

MARV: Marburg virus

MCA: Department of Maternal, Newborn, Child and Adolescent Health (at WHO)

MDA: Ministries, Departments and Agencies

Medevac: Medical evacuation

MERS: Middle East respiratory syndrome

MEURI: Monitored Emergency Use of Unregistered and Investigational Interventions

ML: Money Laundering

MOH: Ministry of Health

MVD: Marburg virus disease

NAPHS: National Action Plan for Health Security

NCDC: Nigeria Centre for Disease Control

NFELTP: Nigeria Field Epidemiology and Laboratory Training Programme

NFP: National Focal Point

NHS: National Health Service (UK)

NHSDPII: National Health Sector Development Plan II

NIH: National Institutes of Health

NPFS: National Pandemic Flu Service

NPHCDA: National Primary Health Care Development Agency

NSAID: non-steroidal anti-inflammatory drug

NSIPSS: National Strategy on Immunization and Primary Health Care Systems Strengthening

OIE: World Organisation for Animal Health / Organisation mondiale de la santé animale

ONSA: Office of the National Security Adviser

OSHA: Occupational Safety and Health Act of 1970 (OSHA)

PECO: population (P), exposure (E), comparator (C), outcome (O)

PHE: Public Health Emergency; Public Health England

PHEIC: Public Health Emergency of International Concern

PHQ-9: Patient health questionnaire 9

PICO: population (P), intervention (I), comparator (C), outcome (O)

PoE: Points of Entry

PPE: personal protective equipment

ProMED: Program for Monitoring Emerging Diseases

PRRS: porcine reproductive and respiratory syndrome

PTSD: Post-traumatic stress disorder

PUD: Peptic ulcer disease

PUI: Persons under investigation

PVS: Performance of Veterinary Systems

RAGIDA: Risk assessment guidelines for infectious diseases transmitted on aircraft

RBA: Risk-Based Approach

RCT: randomized controlled trial

RDT: Rapid diagnostic test

REDISSE: Regional Disease Surveillance Systems Enhancement Project

RHR: Department of Sexual and Reproductive Health and Research (at WHO)

RNA: ribonucleic acid

RRA: Rapid Risk Assessment

RT-PCR: Reverse transcriptase-polymerase chain reaction

RVF: Rift Valley fever

SAGE: Strategic Advisory Group of Experts (SAGE) on Immunization

SARS: Severe acute respiratory syndrome

SDG: Sustainable Development Goals

SFTS: Severe fever with thrombocytopaenia syndrome

SOP: Standard operating procedure

SPAR: State Party Annual Reporting Tool

SRB: Self-Regulating Body

STI: Sexually transmitted infection

TB: Tuberculosis

TF: Terrorist Financing

UN: United Nations

UNFPA: United Nations Population Fund

UNICEF United Nations International Children's Emergency Fund

VHF: Viral haemorrhagic fever

VRAM: Vulnerability Risk Assessment Mapping

WHO: World Health Organization

WPV: Wild Polio Virus

GLOSSARY OF TERMINOLOGY

Cluster

Cluster refers to an aggregation of cases grouped in place and time that are suspected to be greater than the number expected, even though the expected number may not be known. (CDC 2012)

Consequences

Consequences are the negative effects of a disaster expressed in terms of human impacts, economic and environmental impacts, and political/social impacts. (ISO 31010)

Contact

Refers to a person not currently presenting symptoms, who has contact with, or may have been in contact with, a confirmed HCID case, bodily fluids from a case, or the contaminated environment within a period equal to the maximum incubation period. (ECDC 2019)

Contact tracing

The identification and follow-up of persons who may have come into contact with a person infected with a certain pathogen.

Contacts can be offered advice, testing and treatment or immunization depending on their type of exposure. If no treatment or vaccine are available, they can be monitored for a period equal to the maximum incubation period for signs of illness. They may also have to be isolated for the same period of time to prevent ongoing transmission. (ECDC 2019)

EARLY WARNING SYSTEM

A system for identification of potential crises, mainly through bulletins, forecasts, alerts. (ECDC 2019)

ENDEMIC

Endemic refers to the constant presence and/or usual prevalence of a disease or infectious agent in a population within a geographic area. (CDC 2012)

EPIDEMIC

Epidemic refers to an increase, often sudden, in the number of cases of a disease above what is normally expected in that population in that area. Outbreak carries the same definition of epidemic, but is often used for a more limited geographic area. (CDC 2012)

EXPOSURE

People, property, systems, or other elements present in hazard zones that are thereby subject to potential losses. (UNISDR, 2009)

Hazard

Hazard is a dangerous phenomenon, substance, human activity or condition that may cause loss of life, injury or other health impacts, property damage, loss of livelihoods and services, social and economic disruption, or environmental damage. (European Commission 2010)

Hazard assessments

Hazard assessments determine the probability of occurrence of a certain hazard of certain intensity. (European Commission 2010)

Hazard map

Hazard map is a map that portrays levels of probability of a hazard occurring across a geographical area. Such maps can focus on one hazard only or include several types of hazards (multi-hazard map). (European Commission 2010)

High-Consequence Infectious Disease (HCID)

Also known as Infectious Disease of High Consequence (IDHC). HCIDs constitute serious human health threats. Patients with such diseases typically develop severe symptoms and require a high level of care. The case-fatality rates can be high. Several HCIDs are transmissible from person to person and therefore require healthcare workers to take precautions to prevent transmission. (ECDC 2019)

Human impacts

Human impacts are defined as the quantitative measurement of the following factors: number of deaths, number of severely injured or ill people, and number of permanently displaced people. (European Commission 2010)

Hyperendemic

Hyperendemic refers to persistent, high levels of disease occurrence. (CDC 2012)

Influenza Pandemic

An influenza pandemic occurs when a new influenza virus emerges and spreads around the world, and most people do not have immunity. Viruses that have caused past pandemics typically originated from animal influenza viruses. (World Health Organization 2010)

Medical evacuation (medevac)

The evacuation of persons, usually by air transportation, accompanied by trained personnel able to provide care, to a place where they can receive appropriate medical care. In the case of an HCID (probable or confirmed) patient, there is an additional need to mitigate transmission risks during the medevac operation. (ECDC 2019)

MULTI-HAZARD ASSESSMENTS

Multi-hazard assessments determine the likelihood of occurrence of different hazards either occurring at the same time or shortly following each other, because they are dependent from one another or because they are caused by the same triggering event or hazard, or merely threatening the same elements at risk (vulnerable/ exposed elements) without chronological coincidence. (European Commission 2010)

MULTI-HAZARD MAP

Multi-hazard map is a map that portrays levels of probability of several hazards occurring across a geographical area. (European Commission 2010)

MULTI-RISK ASSESSMENTS

Multi-risk assessments determine the total risk from several hazards either occurring at the same time or shortly following each other, because they are dependent from one another or because they are caused by the same triggering event or hazard; or merely threatening the same elements at risk (vulnerable/exposed elements) without chronological coincidence. (European Commission 2010)

NATURAL HAZARD

Natural process or phenomenon that may cause loss of life, injury or other health impacts, property damage, loss of livelihoods and services, social and economic disruption, or environmental damage. (European Commission 2010)

PANDEMIC

A pandemic is the worldwide spread of a new disease. (World Health Organization 2010)

PERSON UNDER INVESTIGATION (PUI)

A term mainly used in the case of Ebola virus disease and refers to a person meeting the clinical and the epidemiological criteria OR a person with history of high-risk exposure and any of the listed symptoms of EVD, including fever of any grade. (ECDC 2019)

POINTS OF ENTRY (POE)

The International Health Regulations (IHR) define a point of entry as 'a passage for international entry or exit of travellers, baggage, cargo, containers, conveyances, goods and postal parcels, as well as agencies and areas providing services to them on entry or exit'. (ECDC 2019)

PREPAREDNESS

The knowledge and capacities developed by government, professional response and recovery organisations, communities and individuals to effectively anticipate, respond to and recover from the impacts of likely, imminent or current crisis. (ECDC 2019)

Preparedness planning

Involves factoring in plans at the local, national and EU level in various sectors that affect emergency plans. Preparedness plans provide a backbone structure for developing core elements to address different types of health threats and improve the interoperability of such plans; preparedness planning addresses threats and emergencies that threaten or are likely to threaten public health in a Member State. (ECDC 2019)

ProMED-mail

ProMED-mail is an internet-based surveillance system that disseminates information on outbreaks of infectious diseases and acute exposures to toxins based on media reports and reports from subscribers. It reports on diseases that affect human health, including those in animals and in plants grown for food or animal feed. (Hitchcock P, Chamberlain A, Van Wagoner M, Inglesby TV, O'Toole T. 2007).

Public health risk

The likelihood of an event that may adversely affect the health of human populations, with an emphasis on whether it may spread internationally or present a serious and direct danger. (ECDC 2019)

Public health threat

An event (incident), condition or agent, which by its presence has the potential to rapidly harm - directly or indirectly - an exposed population in such a way as to lead to a crisis. (ECDC 2019)

Resilience

The ability of a system, community or society exposed to hazards to resist, absorb, accommodate to and recover from the effects of a hazard in a timely and efficient manner, including through the preservation and restoration of its essential basic structures and functions. (UNISDR, 2009)

Response

The provision of emergency services and public assistance during or immediately after a crisis, in order to save lives, reduce impact on health, environment and society, ensure public safety and meet the basic subsistence needs of those affected. (ECDC 2019)

Risk

Risk is the combination of the probability of a crisis and its negative consequences. (ECDC 2019) It can also be defined as a combination of the consequences of an event (hazard) and the associated likelihood/probability of its occurrence. (ISO 31010)

RISK ANALYSIS

Risk analysis is the process to comprehend the nature of risk and to determine the level of risk. (ISO 31010)

RISK ASSESSMENT

A scientifically based process consisting of the following steps: i) hazard identification, ii) hazard characterisation, iii) exposure assessment and iv) risk characterisation. (ECDC 2019)

RISK COMMUNICATION

The exchange and dissemination of adequate information concerning risks to enable decision makers, stakeholders and the public to make appropriate decisions. (ECDC 2019)

RISK CRITERIA

Risk criteria are the terms of reference against which the significance of a risk is evaluated. (ISO 31010)

RISK EVALUATION

Risk evaluation is the process of comparing the results of risk analysis with risk criteria to determine whether the risk and/or its magnitude is acceptable or tolerable. (ISO 31010)

Risk identification

Risk identification is the process of finding, recognizing and describing risks. (ISO 31010)

Risk management

The process, distinct from risk assessment, of weighing policy alternatives, risk assessment and other factors that are relevant for protecting the health of consumers – in consultation with all parties involved. If necessary, this process may result in the selection of appropriate prevention and control options. (ECDC 2019)

Risk map

Risk map is a map that portrays levels of risk across a geographical area. Such maps can focus on one risk only or include different types of risks. (European Commission 2010)

Risk scenario

Risk scenario is a representation of one single-risk or multi-risk situation leading to significant impacts, selected for the purpose of assessing in more detail a particular type of risk for which it is representative, or constitutes an informative example or illustration. (European Commission 2010)

SINGLE-RISK ASSESSMENTS

Single-risk assessments determine the singular risk (i.e. likelihood and consequences) of one particular hazard (e.g. flood) or one particular type of hazard (e.g. flooding) occurring in a particular geographic area during a given period of time. (European Commission 2010)

SPORADIC

Sporadic refers to a disease that occurs infrequently and irregularly. (CDC 2012)

STANDARD OPERATING PROCEDURES (SOP)

Standard Operating Procedures are documents that prescribe the operational steps to be followed in relation to processes or policies, so that they are performed in the same way every time to guarantee the outcome. (ECDC 2019)

SURVEILLANCE

The systematic ongoing collection, collation and analysis of data for public health purposes, combined with the timely dissemination of public health information for assessment and public health response. (ECDC 2019)

TECHNOLOGICAL HAZARD

A hazard originating from technological or industrial conditions, including accidents, dangerous procedures, infrastructure failures or specific human activities, that may cause loss of life, injury, illness or other health impacts, property damage, loss of livelihoods and services, social and economic disruption, or environmental damage. (UNISDR, 2009)

THREAT

Threat is a potentially damaging physical event, phenomenon or activity of an intentional/ malicious character. (European Commission 2010)

VULNERABILITY

The characteristics and circumstances of a community, system or asset that make it susceptible to the damaging effects of a hazard. (UNISDR, 2009)

In probabilistic/quantitative risk assessments the term vulnerability expresses the part or percentage of Exposure that is likely to be lost due to a certain hazard. (European Commission 2010)

WHO GISRS

"WHO GISRS" means the international network of influenza laboratories, coordinated by WHO, that conduct year-round surveillance of influenza, assessing the risk of pandemic influenza and assisting in preparedness measures. The WHO GISRS comprises National Influenza Centres, WHO Collaborating Centres on Influenza, WHO H5 Reference Laboratories and Essential Regulatory Laboratories.

CHAPTER 1

INTRODUCTION TO EMERGING INFECTIOUS DISEASES: STEMMING THE TIDE

Emerging infectious diseases in animals or humans pose a constant threat to human health and life. Some infectious diseases have high mortality and fatality rates, and some of these diseases lack treatments or vaccines.[1] The World Health Organization (WHO) and the Program for Monitoring Emerging Diseases (ProMED)-mail together report more than 3,000 alerts of human infectious diseases annually. Consequently, devoting extraordinary public health resources to tracking and preparing a response must depend on the estimated risk that the outbreak will reach a given jurisdiction and cause widespread, serious illness.[2] Annual changes in host and parasite

---

[1] Liao Y, Xu B, Wang J, Liu X. A new method for assessing the risk of infectious disease outbreak. *Sci Rep*. 2017;7:40084. Published 2017 Jan 9. doi:10.1038/srep40084 (accessed 8 June 2020).

[2] Marc Lipsitch, Lyn Finelli, Richard T. Heffernan, Gabriel M. Leung, and Stephen C. Redd (2011), 'Improving the Evidence Base for Decision Making During a Pandemic: The Example of 2009 Influenza A/H1N1', Biosecurity and Bioterrorism: Biodefense Strategy, Practice, and Science Volume 9, Number 2, Available at: http://doi.org/10.1089/bsp.2011.0007 (accessed 6 June 2020).

biology can generate outbreaks that occur around the same time each year, although it is important to distinguish observed seasonal outbreaks of infectious diseases from seasonal drivers of epidemic parameters. Indeed, in nonlinear systems, response frequencies and driving frequencies need not be the same.[3]

Emerging infectious diseases are broadly defined as infections that have newly appeared in a population or have existed but are rapidly increasing in incidence or geographical range. The classic definition of a pandemic is "an epidemic occurring worldwide, or over a very wide area, crossing international boundaries and usually affecting a large number of people.[4]

Emerging infectious diseases, which include pandemic influenza outbreaks, have risen substantially over time and are dominated by zoonoses (60%) of which most (72%) originate in wildlife. Emergence occurs at the human–animal interface, when animal infections breach species barriers to infect human beings, the population in which they are often first identified. In many instances identification occurs many years after the breach.[5]

---

[3] Altizer S, Dobson A, Hosseini P, Hudson P, Pascual M, Rohani P. Seasonality and the dynamics of infectious diseases. *Ecol Lett.* 2006;9(4):467-484. doi:10.1111/j.1461-0248.2005.00879.x (accessed 6 June 2020).

[4] McCloskey B, Dar O, Zumla A, Heymann DL. Emerging infectious diseases and pandemic potential: status quo and reducing risk of global spread. *Lancet Infect Dis.* 2014;14(10):1001-1010. doi:10.1016/S1473-3099(14)70846-1 (accessed 9 June 2020).

[5] McCloskey B, Dar O, Zumla A, Heymann DL. Emerging infectious diseases and pandemic potential: status quo and reducing risk of global spread. *Lancet Infect Dis.*

Coping with, and trying to understand, emerging epidemics has been part of the human experience since time immemorial. The concern that attends the emergence of a novel infectious disease might be substantial, but fears often subside as the disease becomes better understood, partly because initial findings tend to be biased towards cases and case clusters with more severe outcomes.[6]

1.1. EMERGING INFECTIOUS DISEASES THAT HAVE BEEN IDENTIFIED IN THE PAST 40 YEARS

During the past 40 years, emerging infectious diseases that have been identified range from coronavirus disease 2019 (COVID-19), Middle East respiratory syndrome, severe acute respiratory syndrome, and Ebola, to Marburg haemorrhagic fever, avian influenza, seasonal influenza, pandemic influenza, and human immunodeficiency virus (HIV).[7]

This section will expound on the aforementioned infectious diseases with a focus on their definition, history, symptoms,

2014;14(10):1001-1010. doi:10.1016/S1473-3099(14)70846-1 (accessed 9 June 2020).

[6] David N Fisman and Ashleigh R Tuite (2014), 'The epidemiology of MERS-CoV', THE LANCET Infectious Diseases, VOLUME 14, ISSUE 1, P6-7, Available at: https://www.thelancet.com/journals/laninf/article/PIIS1473-3099(13)70283-4/fulltext (accessed 6 June 2020).

[7] McCloskey B, Dar O, Zumla A, Heymann DL. Emerging infectious diseases and pandemic potential: status quo and reducing risk of global spread. *Lancet Infect Dis.* 2014;14(10):1001-1010. doi:10.1016/S1473-3099(14)70846-1

transmission, incubation period, diagnosis, treatment, and prevention.

1.1.1. COVID-19

COVID-19 is the infectious disease caused by the most recently discovered coronavirus - SARS-CoV-2.[8] This new virus and disease were unknown before the outbreak began in Wuhan, China, in December 2019.[9] The disease spreads from person to person through infected air droplets that are projected during sneezing or coughing. It can also be transmitted when humans have contact with hands or surfaces that contain the virus and touch their eyes, nose, or mouth with the contaminated hands. COVID-19 was first reported in China, but it has now spread throughout the world.[10]

People with COVID-19 have had a wide range of symptoms reported – ranging from mild symptoms to severe illness. Symptoms may appear 2-14 days after exposure to the virus. People with these symptoms may have COVID-19:

- Fever or chills

---

[8] JOHN HOPKINS MEDICINE (2020), 'What Is Coronavirus?', Available at: https://www.hopkinsmedicine.org/health/conditions-and-diseases/coronavirus (accessed 30 May 2020).
[9] World Health Organization (2020), 'Q&A on coronaviruses (COVID-19)', Available at: https://www.who.int/emergencies/diseases/novel-coronavirus-2019/question-and-answers-hub/q-a-detail/q-a-coronaviruses (accessed 26 July 2020).
[10] Africa Centres for Disease Control and Prevention (Africa CDC) (2020), 'Coronavirus Disease 2019 (COVID-19)', Available at: https://africacdc.org/covid-19/ (accessed 26 July 2020).

- Cough
- Shortness of breath or difficulty breathing
- Fatigue
- Muscle or body aches
- Headache
- New loss of taste or smell
- Sore throat
- Congestion or runny nose
- Nausea or vomiting
- Diarrhea.[11]

To reduce the risk of infection or spread of COVID-19, members of the public are advised to adhere to the following hand and respiratory hygiene measures:

- Wash your hands regularly with soap and water or use an alcohol-based sanitiser if no water and soap is available.
- Use a non-medical face mask/covering for all persons while in public spaces.
- Practice no-touch greetings.
- Maintain at least 2 metres physical distance between yourself and anyone who is coughing or sneezing.

[11] United States Centers for Disease Control and Prevention (2020), 'Symptoms of Coronavirus', Available at: https://www.cdc.gov/coronavirus/2019-ncov/symptoms-testing/symptoms.html (accessed 26 July 2020).

- Avoid crowded spaces such as open markets, crowded supermarkets and pharmacies.
- Adhere to other national and state directives.[12]

1.1.2. MIDDLE EAST RESPIRATORY SYNDROME (MERS)

Middle East respiratory syndrome (MERS) is a viral respiratory illness caused by a coronavirus (Middle East respiratory syndrome coronavirus, or MERS-CoV) that was first identified in Saudi Arabia in 2012. Coronaviruses are a large family of viruses that can cause diseases in humans, ranging from the common cold to Severe Acute Respiratory Syndrome (SARS).[13]

Though the animal to human route is not fully understood, dromedary camels are a major host for MERS-CoV, and direct or indirect contact with an infected animal may lead to transmission. Human to human cases are limited so far, but have occurred among family members, patients, and healthcare workers in very close contact. A majority of cases of the virus

---

[12] Nigeria Centre for Disease Control (2020), 'Frequently Asked Questions on Coronavirus', Available at: https://covid19.ncdc.gov.ng/faq/ (accessed 27 August 2020).

[13] World Health Organization (2019), 'Frequently asked questions on Middle East respiratory syndrome coronavirus (MERS-CoV)', Available at: https://www.who.int/csr/disease/coronavirus_infections/faq/en/ (accessed 3rd of August 2020).

have been transmitted in healthcare settings before MERS-CoV was diagnosed.[14]

The clinical spectrum of MERS-CoV infection ranges from no symptoms (asymptomatic) or mild respiratory symptoms to severe acute respiratory disease and death. A typical presentation of MERS-CoV disease is fever, cough and shortness of breath. Pneumonia is a common finding, but not always present. Gastrointestinal symptoms, including diarrhoea, have also been reported. Severe illness can cause respiratory failure that requires mechanical ventilation and support in an intensive care unit. The virus appears to cause more severe disease in older people, people with weakened immune systems, and those with chronic diseases such as renal disease, cancer, chronic lung disease, and diabetes.[15]

Infection prevention and control measures are critical to prevent the possible spread of MERS-CoV in health care facilities. It is not always possible to identify patients with MERS-CoV infection early because like other respiratory infections, the early symptoms of MERS-CoV infection are non-specific. Therefore, healthcare workers should always apply

---

[14] Africa Centres for Disease Control and Prevention (Africa CDC) (2020), 'Middle East Respiratory Syndrome', Available at: https://africacdc.org/disease/middle-east-respiratory-syndrome/ (accessed 6 September 2020).

[15] World Health Organization (2019), 'Middle East respiratory syndrome coronavirus (MERS-CoV)', Available at: https://www.who.int/en/news-room/fact-sheets/detail/middle-east-respiratory-syndrome-coronavirus-(mers-cov) (accessed 4th of August 2020).

standard precautions consistently with all patients, regardless of their diagnosis. Droplet precautions should be added to the standard precautions when providing care to patients with symptoms of acute respiratory infection; contact precautions and eye protection should be added when caring for probable or confirmed cases of MERS-CoV infection; airborne precautions should be applied when performing aerosol generating procedures.[16]

Supportive therapies prevent complications and increase chances of survival. They include: oxygen, antimicrobials, specific treatment for underlying conditions such as diabetes, kidney failure, etc. Treatment is based on a person's clinical condition.[17]

No vaccine or specific treatment for MERS is currently available, however there are several vaccines for MERS in development. Treatment is supportive and based on a person's clinical condition.[18]

---

[16] World Health Organization (2019), 'Middle East respiratory syndrome coronavirus (MERS-CoV) – The Kingdom of Saudi Arabia', Available at: https://www.who.int/csr/don/05-december-2019-mers-saudi-arabia/en/ (accessed 3rd of August 2020).

[17] World Health Organization. (2018). Managing epidemics: key facts about major deadly diseases. World Health Organization. https://apps.who.int/iris/handle/10665/272442. License: CC BY-NC-SA 3.0 IGO (accessed 4th of August 2020).

[18] World Health Organization (2019), 'Frequently asked questions on Middle East respiratory syndrome coronavirus (MERS-CoV)', Available at: https://www.who.int/csr/disease/coronavirus_infections/faq/en/ (accessed 3rd of August 2020).

1.1.3. SEVERE ACUTE RESPIRATORY SYNDROME (SARS)

Severe acute respiratory syndrome (SARS) is a viral respiratory illness caused by a coronavirus called SARS-associated coronavirus (SARS-CoV). SARS was first reported in Asia in February 2003. The illness spread to more than two dozen countries in North America, South America, Europe, and Asia before the SARS global outbreak of 2003 was contained.[19]

The main way that SARS seems to spread is by close person-to-person contact. The virus that causes SARS is thought to be transmitted most readily by respiratory droplets (droplet spread) produced when an infected person coughs or sneezes. Droplet spread can happen when droplets from the cough or sneeze of an infected person are propelled a short distance (generally up to 3 feet) through the air and deposited on the mucous membranes of the mouth, nose, or eyes of persons who are nearby. The virus also can spread when a person touches a surface or object contaminated with infectious droplets and then touches his or her mouth, nose, or eye(s). In addition, it is possible that the

[19] United States Centers for Disease Control and Prevention (2017), 'Severe Acute Respiratory Syndrome (SARS)', Available at: https://www.cdc.gov/sars/index.html (accessed 26 July 2020).

SARS virus might spread more broadly through the air (airborne spread) or by other ways that are not now known.[20]

In general, SARS begins with a high fever (temperature greater than 100.4°F [>38.0°C]). Other symptoms may include headache, an overall feeling of discomfort, and body aches. Some people also have mild respiratory symptoms at the outset. About 10 percent to 20 percent of patients have diarrhea. After 2 to 7 days, SARS patients may develop a dry cough. Most patients develop pneumonia.[21]

During the 2003 epidemic, the community containment strategy for the United States consisted mainly of coordinating SARS response activities through the Centers for Disease Control and Prevention's Emergency Operations Center and providing information and education to the public, healthcare workers, and others. Activities included issuing guidelines and fact sheets, holding press conferences, and meeting with groups and communities to address their concerns about stigmatization. The Centers for Disease Control and Prevention (CDC) also recommended isolation of SARS patients until they were believed to be no longer infectious. This practice allowed patients to receive appropriate care and helped contain the

---

20 United States Centers for Disease Control and Prevention (2017), 'SARS Basics Fact Sheet', Available at: https://www.cdc.gov/sars/about/fs-sars.html (accessed 26 July 2020).

21 United States Centers for Disease Control and Prevention (2017), 'SARS Basics Fact Sheet', Available at: https://www.cdc.gov/sars/about/fs-sars.html (accessed 26 July 2020).

spread of infection. Severely ill persons were cared for in hospitals; those with mild illnesses were cared for at home. Sick persons in home isolation were asked to avoid contact with others and to remain at home until 10 days after the resolution of fever, provided respiratory symptoms were absent or improving. In the United States, where there was little or no transmission of SARS-CoV, neither individual nor population-based quarantine of contacts was recommended. CDC advised persons who were exposed but not symptomatic to monitor themselves for symptoms and advised home isolation and medical evaluation if symptoms appeared.[22]

1.1.4. EBOLA VIRUS DISEASE

Ebola virus disease (EVD) is a viral hemorrhagic fever with a high mortality rate.[23] EVD was first identified in Zaire in 1976 and there have since been at least twenty-five outbreaks in Africa. The 2014 West African outbreak—first reported in Guinea and subsequently becoming established in Liberia and Sierra Leone—is the largest to date.[24] Infections with Ebola viruses

---

[22] United States Centers for Disease Control and Prevention (2004), 'Public Health Guidance for Community-Level Preparedness and Response to Severe Acute Respiratory Syndrome (SARS) Version 2', Available at: https://www.cdc.gov/sars/guidance/i-infection/index.html (accessed 26 July 2020).

[23] Riad, M.H., Sekamatte, M., Ocom, F. *et al.* Risk assessment of Ebola virus disease spreading in Uganda using a two-layer temporal network. *Sci Rep* **9,** 16060 (2019). https://doi.org/10.1038/s41598-019-52501-1 (accessed 26 July 2020).

[24] Moss R, Hickson RI, McVernon J, McCaw JM, Hort K, Black J, et al. (2016) Model-Informed Risk Assessment and Decision Making for an Emerging

originating from Africa cause a severe disease in humans called Ebola virus disease.[25]

There are five species of the genus Ebolavirus (Filoviridae family): Zaire ebolavirus, Sudan ebolavirus, Reston ebolavirus, Tai Forest ebolavirus, and Bundibugyo ebolavirus. Ebola viruses are biosafety level-4 pathogens (BSL-4, risk group 4) and require special containment measures and barrier protection, particularly for healthcare workers.[26] All five species are found in Africa and cause serious illness in humans. In addition, Reston virus, species Reston ebolavirus (RESTV) can cause epizootics reported in the Philippines and China, but Reston virus only causes asymptomatic infection in humans. The Marburgvirus genus contains only one species, Marburg marburgvirus (MARV), which is responsible for several outbreaks of haemorrhagic fever in Africa. The Cuevavirus genus of the Filoviridae family contains the Lloviu cuevavirus, another filovirus detected in European bats. Recently, two new bat filovirus species were proposed within the Filoviridae family: the

Infectious Disease in the Asia-Pacific Region. PLoS Negl Trop Dis 10(9): e0005018. https://doi.org/10.1371/journal.pntd.0005018 (accessed 26 July 2020).

25 European Centre for Disease Prevention and Control. Rapid risk assessment: Ebola virus disease outbreak in North Kivu and Ituri Provinces, Democratic Republic of the Congo – 9 August 2018. Stockholm: ECDC, 2018. Available from: http://ecdc.europa.eu/publications-data/rapid-risk-assessment-ebola-virus-disease-outbreak-north-kivu-and-ituri-provinces

26 European Centre for Disease Prevention and Control. Rapid risk assessment: Ebola virus disease outbreak in North Kivu and Ituri Provinces, Democratic Republic of the Congo – 9 August 2018. Stockholm: ECDC, 2018. Available from: http://ecdc.europa.eu/publications-data/rapid-risk-assessment-ebola-virus-disease-outbreak-north-kivu-and-ituri-provinces

Bombali virus, species Bombali ebolavirus (BOMV) found in little free-tailed bats (Chaerephon pumilus) and in Angola free-tailed bats (Mops condylurus) in Bombali District, Sierra Leone and the Měnglà virus, species Mengla dianlovirus (MLAV) identified in liver tissue of a bat (genus Rousettus) from Mengla County, Yunnan Province, China. To date, these viruses are not known to be pathogenic for humans. Further genera of the Filoviridae family (Striavirus genus and Thamnovirus genus) contain filoviruses detected in fishes.[27]

The incubation period is usually four to ten days but can be as short as two days and as long as 21 days. The symptoms usually consist of a sudden onset of fever, malaise, headache, muscle pain and sore throat. This phase can be followed by symptoms and clinical manifestations from several organ systems (gastrointestinal, neurological, vascular, cutaneous and respiratory). Severe exhaustion, haemorrhagic manifestations and multi-organ failure occur in the severe form of EVD. The case–fatality ratio for *Zaire ebolavirus* infections is estimated to be between 44% and 90%.[28]

---

[27] European Centre for Disease Prevention and Control. Factsheet about Ebola and Marburg fevers [Internet]. Stockholm: ECDC; 2016 [cited 11 April 2019]. Available from: http://ecdc.europa.eu/ebola-and-marburg-fevers/facts/factsheet (accessed 8 August 2020).

[28] European Centre for Disease Prevention and Control. Rapid risk assessment: Ebola virus disease outbreak in North Kivu and Ituri Provinces, Democratic Republic of the Congo – first update – 4 October 2018. Stockholm: ECDC, 2018. Available from: http://ecdc.europa.eu/publications-data/rapid-risk-assessment-ebola-virus-disease-outbreak-north-kivu-and-ituri-first-update (accessed 8 August 2020).

Ebola viruses are highly transmissible through direct contact with infected blood, secretions, tissues, organs and other bodily fluids from dead or living infected animals or persons. Transmission through infected semen from a male survivor to his female partner has been reported. Transmission via objects contaminated with infected bodily fluids (fomites) is possible. The principal mode of transmission in outbreaks among humans is person-to-person through direct contact with symptomatic or dead cases. Airborne transmission has not been documented. The risk of transmission is low in the early phase of human disease.[29] The risk of a traveller becoming infected with Ebola virus during a visit to the affected areas and developing disease after returning is extremely low, even if the visit included travel to areas where primary cases have been reported. Transmission, as stated earlier, requires direct contact with blood, secretions, other body fluid or tissues of infected persons, or with infected dead bodies or animals, all unlikely exposures for the average traveller. Travellers are strongly advised to avoid all such contacts. The risk for travellers visiting family and friends in affected areas is similarly low, unless the traveller has direct physical contact with a sick or dead person or animal infected

---

29 European Centre for Disease Prevention and Control. Rapid risk assessment: Ebola virus disease outbreak in North Kivu and Ituri Provinces, Democratic Republic of the Congo – second update – 21 December 2018. Stockholm: ECDC, 2018. Available from: http://ecdc.europa.eu/publications-data/rapid-risk-assessment-ebola-outbreak-north-kivu-and-ituri-second-update (accessed 8 August 2020).

with Ebola virus. Visitors are strongly advised to avoid all direct physical contact with a sick or dead person infected with Ebola virus. There is a risk for health care workers and volunteers, especially if involved in caring for EVD patients. The risk can be considered low, unless adequate infection prevention and control measures (such as use of clean water and soap or alcohol-based hand rubs, personal protective equipment, safe injection practices and proper waste management) are not followed, including at medical services at ports, airports and ground crossings.[30]

In most cases, an infected patient experiences a sudden onset of flu-like illness, with fever, general malaise and weakness, muscle and joint pains and headache, followed by progressive weakness, anorexia, diarrhoea (watery stools sometimes containing blood and mucus), nausea and vomiting. This first set of symptoms corresponds to the prodromal phase (duration up to 10 days). The next stage of the disease is characterised by symptoms and clinical manifestations from several organ systems. Symptoms can be gastrointestinal (vomiting, diarrhoea, anorexia and abdominal pain), neurological (headaches, confusion), vascular (conjunctival/pharyngeal injections), cutaneous (maculopapular rash) and respiratory (cough, chest

[30] World Health Organization (2014), 'Travel and transport risk assessment: Interim guidance for public health authorities and the transport sector', Available at: https://www.who.int/csr/resources/publications/ebola/travel-guidance/en/ (accessed 24 July 2020).

pain, shortness of breath) and can include complete exhaustion (prostration). Haemorrhagic manifestations can appear (e.g. bloody diarrhoea, nosebleeds, haematemesis, petechiae, ecchymoses and prolonged bleeding from needle puncture sites). Certain patients develop profuse internal and external haemorrhages and disseminated intravascular coagulation. Patients in the final stage of disease die from a combination of multi-organ failure and hypovolemic shock due to severe fluid losses. Case fatality rates (CFR) vary according to the species of Ebola virus, with ZEBOV exhibiting higher fatality. Based on one literature review, the weighted CFR for Ebola virus disease was assessed to be 65.0% [95% CI (54.0–76.0%)].[31]

Ebola virus is known to persist in immune-privileged sites in some people who have recovered from Ebola virus disease. These sites include the testicles, the inside of the eye, and the central nervous system. In women who have been infected while pregnant, the virus persists in the placenta, amniotic fluid and fetus. In women who have been infected while breastfeeding, the virus may persist in breast milk. Relapse-symptomatic illness in someone who has recovered from EVD due to increased replication of the virus in a specific site is a rare event, but has been documented. Reasons for this phenomenon are not yet

[31] European Centre for Disease Prevention and Control. Factsheet about Ebola and Marburg fevers [Internet]. Stockholm: ECDC; 2016 [cited 11 April 2019]. Available from: http://ecdc.europa.eu/ebola-and-marburg-fevers/facts/factsheet (accessed 8 August 2020).

fully understood. Studies of viral persistence indicate that in a small percentage of survivors, some body fluids may test positive on a real-time reverse transcription polymerase chain reaction (RT-PCR) testing for Ebola virus for longer than 9 months. More surveillance data and research are needed on the risks of sexual transmission, and particularly on the prevalence of viable and transmissible virus in semen over time.[32]

Community engagement is key to successfully controlling outbreaks. Raising awareness of risk factors for Ebola infection and protective measures (including vaccination) that individuals can take is an effective way to reduce human transmission.[33] Supportive care - rehydration with oral or intravenous fluids - and treatment of specific symptoms improves survival. There is as yet no proven treatment available for EVD. However, a range of potential treatments including blood products, immune therapies and drug therapies are currently being evaluated.[34]

An experimental Ebola vaccine proved highly protective against EVD in a major trial in Guinea in 2015. The vaccine, called rVSV-ZEBOV, was studied in a trial involving 11 841

---

[32] World Health Organization. Ebola virus disease [Internet]. Geneva: WHO; 2019 [cited 11 April 2019]. Available from: http://www.who.int/news-room/fact-sheets/detail/ebola-virus-disease

[33] World Health Organization (2020), 'Ebola virus disease', Available at: https://www.who.int/en/news-room/fact-sheets/detail/ebola-virus-disease (accessed 4th of August 2020).

[34] World Health Organization (2020), 'Ebola virus disease', Available at: https://www.who.int/en/news-room/fact-sheets/detail/ebola-virus-disease (accessed 4th of August 2020).

people. Among the 5837 people who received the vaccine, no Ebola cases were recorded 10 days or more after vaccination. In comparison, there were 23 cases 10 days or more after vaccination among those who did not receive the vaccine.[35]

1.1.5. MARBURG VIRUS DISEASE

Marburg virus is the causative agent of Marburg virus disease (MVD), a disease with a case fatality ratio of up to 88%.[36] Marburg virus was first recognized in 1967, when outbreaks of hemorrhagic fever occurred simultaneously in laboratories in Marburg and Frankfurt, Germany and in Belgrade, Yugoslavia (now Serbia). Thirty-one people became ill, initially laboratory workers followed by several medical personnel and family members who had cared for them. Seven deaths were reported. The first people infected had been exposed to imported African green monkeys or their tissues while conducting research. One additional case was diagnosed retrospectively.[37]

Marburg and Ebola viruses are both members of the Filoviridae family (filovirus). Though caused by different

---

[35] World Health Organization (2020), 'Ebola virus disease', Available at: https://www.who.int/en/news-room/fact-sheets/detail/ebola-virus-disease (accessed 4th of August 2020).

[36] World Health Organization (2018), 'Marburg virus disease', Available at: https://www.who.int/news-room/fact-sheets/detail/marburg-virus-disease (accessed 28 July 2020).

[37] United States Centers for Disease Control and Prevention (2014), 'Marburg hemorrhagic fever (Marburg HF)', Available at: https://www.cdc.gov/vhf/marburg/index.html (accessed 28 July 2020).

viruses, the two diseases are clinically similar. Both diseases are rare and have the capacity to cause dramatic outbreaks with high fatality rates.[38] Marburg viruses are highly transmissible by direct contact (e.g. through mucous membranes or broken skin) with blood, other bodily fluids (e.g. saliva, urine, vomit) of living or dead infected persons or any surfaces and materials soiled by infectious fluids. Transmission can also occur by contact with dead or living infected animals, including bushmeat (e.g. monkeys, chimpanzees, forest antelopes and bats) or by visiting caves or mines colonised by bats. Marburg viruses can persist in immune-privileged sites of certain survivors such as testicles, central nervous system and aqueous humour from which new transmissions can potentially arise, notably through sexual transmission.[39]

Marburg virus disease has an incubation period ranging from 2–21 days (usually 5–10 days). The disease is characterized by a sudden onset of high fever, headache and general malaise. Gastrointestinal symptoms usually appear by the third day (nausea, vomiting, abdominal pain and watery diarrhoea). Approximately five to seven days after the onset of symptoms, patients may exhibit a maculopapular non-itchy rash mostly on

---

[38] World Health Organization (2018), 'Marburg virus disease', Available at: https://www.who.int/news-room/fact-sheets/detail/marburg-virus-disease (accessed 28 July 2020).

[39] European Centre for Disease Prevention and Control. Factsheet about Ebola and Marburg fevers [Internet]. Stockholm: ECDC; 2016 [cited 11 April 2019]. Available from: http://ecdc.europa.eu/ebola-and-marburg-fevers/facts/factsheet (accessed 8 August 2020).

their trunk. In severe cases, the central nervous system is involved with confusion, irritability or decreased level of consciousness. Severe haemorrhagic manifestations are observed in many patients. A weighted CFR of 53.8% [95% CI (26.0–80.0%)] has been estimated for Marburg virus disease, but with substantial heterogeneity across outbreaks.[40]

Supportive care – rehydration with oral or intravenous fluids – and treatment of specific symptoms, improves survival. There is as yet no proven treatment available for MVD. However, a range of potential treatments including blood products, immune therapies and drug therapies are currently being evaluated.[41]

1.1.6. AVIAN AND OTHER ZOONOTIC INFLUENZA

Avian influenza is an acute viral disease of the respiratory tract. It is one of several severe zoonotic diseases with pandemic potential in the presence of sustained human-to-human transmission.[42] After an outbreak of A(H5N1) virus in 1997 in poultry in Hong Kong SAR, China, since 2003, this avian and

---

[40] European Centre for Disease Prevention and Control. Factsheet about Ebola and Marburg fevers [Internet]. Stockholm: ECDC; 2016 [cited 11 April 2019]. Available from: http://ecdc.europa.eu/ebola-and-marburg-fevers/facts/factsheet (accessed 8 August 2020).

[41] World Health Organization (2018), 'Marburg virus disease', Available at: https://www.who.int/news-room/fact-sheets/detail/marburg-virus-disease (accessed 28 July 2020).

[42] World Health Organization (2020), 'Avian and other zoonotic influenza: Introduction', Available at: https://openwho.org/courses/avian-and-other-zoonotic-influenza-introduction (accessed 2nd of August 2020).

other influenza viruses have spread from Asia to Europe and Africa. In 2013, human infections with the influenza A(H7N9) virus were reported in China.[43]

There are four types of influenza viruses: types A, B, C and D:

- Influenza A viruses infect humans and many different animals. The emergence of a new and very different influenza A virus with the ability infect people and have sustained human to human transmission, can cause an influenza pandemic.
- Influenza B viruses circulates among humans and cause seasonal epidemics. Recent data showed seals also can be infected.
- Influenza C viruses can infect both humans and pigs but infections are generally mild and are rarely reported.
- Influenza D viruses primarily affect cattle and are not known to infect or cause illness in people.[44]

Influenza type A viruses are of most significance to public health due to their potential to cause an influenza pandemic. Influenza type A viruses are classified into subtypes according to

[43] World Health Organization (2020), 'Avian and other zoonotic influenza', Available at: https://www.who.int/influenza/human_animal_interface/en/ (accessed 2nd of August 2020).

[44] World Health Organization (2018), 'Influenza (Avian and other zoonotic)', Available at: https://www.who.int/en/news-room/fact-sheets/detail/influenza-(avian-and-other-zoonotic) (accessed 2nd of August 2020).

the combinations of different virus surface proteins hemagglutinin (HA) and neuraminidase (NA). So far there are 18 different hemagglutinin subtypes and 11 different neuraminidase subtypes. Depending on the origin host, influenza A viruses can be classified as avian influenza, swine influenza, or other types of animal influenza viruses. Examples include avian influenza "bird flu" virus subtypes A(H5N1) and A(H9N2) or swine influenza "swine flu" virus subtypes A(H1N1) and A(H3N2). All of these animal influenza type A viruses are distinct from human influenza viruses and do not easily transmit among humans.[45]

Aquatic birds are the primary natural reservoir for most subtypes of influenza A viruses. Most cause asymptomatic or mild infection in birds, where the range of symptoms depends on the virus properties. Viruses that cause severe disease in poultry and result in high death rates are called highly pathogenic avian influenza (HPAI). Viruses that cause mild disease in poultry are called low pathogenic avian influenza (LPAI).[46] Most avian influenza viruses do not cause disease in humans, or cause only mild illness, such as fever or conjunctivitis. A few avian influenza viruses are known to cause

---

[45] World Health Organization (2018), 'Influenza (Avian and other zoonotic)', Available at: https://www.who.int/en/news-room/fact-sheets/detail/influenza-(avian-and-other-zoonotic) (accessed 2nd of August 2020).

[46] World Health Organization (2018), 'Influenza (Avian and other zoonotic)', Available at: https://www.who.int/en/news-room/fact-sheets/detail/influenza-(avian-and-other-zoonotic) (accessed 2nd of August 2020).

severe disease with mortality in humans, notably, A(H5N1) and A(H7N9).[47] Disease features such as the incubation period, severity of symptoms and clinical outcome varies by the virus causing infection but mainly manifests with respiratory symptoms.[48]

In terms of transmission, avian influenza viruses can be transmitted directly from wild birds to domestic poultry or indirectly e.g. through contaminated material. The virus spreads directly from bird to bird via airborne transmission or indirectly, through faecal contamination of footwear or feed. Humans are usually infected through close contact with infected birds. Birds shed influenza virus in their faeces and therefore contact with bird droppings is also a possible transmission route.[49]

Avian flu virus is killed by heat and common disinfectants. Thorough cooking of any poultry meat will destroy the virus. The best protective measure is to avoid direct contact with live poultry. Visits to live bird markets and similar places with large

---

[47] European Centre for Disease Prevention and Control, 'Questions and answers on avian influenza', Available at: https://www.ecdc.europa.eu/en/zoonotic-influenza/facts/faq-avian-influenza (accessed 25 August 2020).

[48] World Health Organization (2018), 'Influenza (Avian and other zoonotic)', Available at: https://www.who.int/en/news-room/fact-sheets/detail/influenza-(avian-and-other-zoonotic) (accessed 2nd of August 2020).

[49] European Centre for Disease Prevention and Control, 'Questions and answers on avian influenza', Available at: https://www.ecdc.europa.eu/en/zoonotic-influenza/facts/faq-avian-influenza (accessed 25 August 2020).

concentrations of birds should be avoided, especially in affected areas of Asia.[50]

There is no single vaccine against avian influenza. A specific vaccine is needed for each specific avian influenza strain, and they need to be adapted as the virus continues to change. WHO has suggested candidate vaccine viruses for particular avian reference viruses belonging to different phylogenetic clades for pandemic preparedness.[51]

1.1.7. SEASONAL INFLUENZA

Seasonal influenza is a preventable infectious disease with mostly respiratory symptoms. It is caused by influenza virus and is easily transmitted, predominantly via the droplet and contact routes and by indirect spread from respiratory secretions on hands, tissues, etc. Additionally, aerosol transmission plays a part in influenza virus transmission.[52]

There are 4 types of seasonal influenza viruses, types A, B, C and D. Influenza A and B viruses circulate and cause seasonal epidemics of disease.

---

50 European Centre for Disease Prevention and Control, 'Questions and answers on avian influenza', Available at: https://www.ecdc.europa.eu/en/zoonotic-influenza/facts/faq-avian-influenza (accessed 25 August 2020).

51 European Centre for Disease Prevention and Control, 'Questions and answers on avian influenza', Available at: https://www.ecdc.europa.eu/en/zoonotic-influenza/facts/faq-avian-influenza (accessed 25 August 2020).

52 European Centre for Disease Prevention and Control, 'Factsheet about seasonal influenza', Available at: https://www.ecdc.europa.eu/en/seasonal-influenza/facts/factsheet (accessed 25 August 2020).

- **Influenza A viruses** are further classified into subtypes according to the combinations of the hemagglutinin (HA) and the neuraminidase (NA), the proteins on the surface of the virus. Currently circulating in humans are subtype A(H1N1) and A(H3N2) influenza viruses. The A(H1N1) is also written as A(H1N1)pdm09 as it caused the pandemic in 2009 and subsequently replaced the seasonal influenza A(H1N1) virus which had circulated prior to 2009. Only influenza type A viruses are known to have caused pandemics.
- **Influenza B viruses** are not classified into subtypes, but can be broken down into lineages. Currently circulating influenza type B viruses belong to either B/Yamagata or B/Victoria lineage.
- **Influenza C virus** is detected less frequently and usually causes mild infections, thus does not present public health importance.
- **Influenza D viruses** primarily affect cattle and are not known to infect or cause illness in people.[53]

[53] World Health Organization (2018), 'Influenza (Seasonal)', Available at: https://www.who.int/en/news-room/fact-sheets/detail/influenza-(seasonal) (accessed 2nd of August 2020).

Uncomplicated seasonal influenza disease presents as rapid onset of the following combination of systemic and respiratory symptoms:

- fever or feverishness;
- headache;
- muscle pain;
- general feeling of ill-health;
- runny nose;
- sore throat;
- non-productive cough.[54]

In some cases the disease becomes more severe due to the influenza virus infection or a secondary, usually bacterial, infection e.g. by Streptococcus pneumoniae or Staphylococcus aureus. This most commonly manifests itself in pneumonia, and at times even death. Severe disease may also include myocarditis or encephalitis, which may be fatal. However, quite often the initial influenza infection is not recognised and the death is not classified as being due to influenza. Overall influenza-associated mortality has been estimated to 13.8 per 100,000 person-years (Thompson, 2003).[55]

54 European Centre for Disease Prevention and Control, 'Factsheet about seasonal influenza', Available at: https://www.ecdc.europa.eu/en/seasonal-influenza/facts/factsheet (accessed 25 August 2020).

55 European Centre for Disease Prevention and Control, 'Factsheet about seasonal influenza', Available at: https://www.ecdc.europa.eu/en/seasonal-influenza/facts/factsheet (accessed 25 August 2020).

The elderly on average have a greater risk of developing severe complications, such as pneumonia. They frequently have underlying diseases which reduce their resistance to infection, and their immune response may also be less effective. The young have an increased risk of being infected because they have not developed immunity to the virus. Apart from the age-related increased risk, the risk of complications is increased for people of any age with particular chronic medical conditions:

- metabolic diseases (e.g. diabetes);
- chronic lung conditions (e.g. chronic bronchitis);
- cardiovascular disease (e.g. coronary artery disease);
- hepatic disease;
- haematologic conditions;
- morbid obesity (body mass index >40);
- genetic conditions;
- chronic kidney diseases (e.g. chronic renal failure);
- chronic neurological conditions and physical handicap (e.g. cerebral palsy); and
- conditions and treatments that suppress the immune function (e.g. chemotherapy).[56]

[56] European Centre for Disease Prevention and Control, 'Factsheet about seasonal influenza', Available at: https://www.ecdc.europa.eu/en/seasonal-influenza/facts/factsheet (accessed 25 August 2020).

Moreover, healthy pregnant women have been found to be at increased risk of becoming hospitalized due to respiratory illness during influenza seasons.[57]

In terms of transmission, seasonal influenza spreads easily, with rapid transmission in crowded areas including schools and nursing homes. When an infected person coughs or sneezes, droplets containing viruses (infectious droplets) are dispersed into the air and can spread up to one meter, and infect persons in close proximity who breathe these droplets in. The virus can also be spread by hands contaminated with influenza viruses. To prevent transmission, people should cover their mouth and nose with a tissue when coughing, and wash their hands regularly.[58]

The majority of cases of human influenza are clinically diagnosed. However, during periods of low influenza activity and outside of epidemics situations, the infection of other respiratory viruses e.g. rhinovirus, respiratory syncytial virus, parainfluenza and adenovirus can also present as Influenza-like Illness (ILI) which makes the clinical differentiation of influenza from other pathogens difficult.[59]

---

57 European Centre for Disease Prevention and Control, 'Factsheet about seasonal influenza', Available at: https://www.ecdc.europa.eu/en/seasonal-influenza/facts/factsheet (accessed 25 August 2020).

58 World Health Organization (2018), 'Influenza (Seasonal)', Available at: https://www.who.int/en/news-room/fact-sheets/detail/influenza-(seasonal) (accessed 2nd of August 2020).

59 World Health Organization (2018), 'Influenza (Seasonal)', Available at: https://www.who.int/en/news-room/fact-sheets/detail/influenza-(seasonal) (accessed 2nd of August 2020).

Patients that are not from a high-risk group should be managed with symptomatic treatment and are advised, if symptomatic, to stay home in order to minimize the risk of infecting others in the community. Treatment focuses on relieving symptoms of influenza such as fever. Patients should monitor themselves to detect if their condition deteriorates and seek medical attention Patients that are known to be in a group at high risk for developing severe or complicated illness, (see above) should be treated with antivirals in addition to symptomatic treatment as soon as possible.

Patients with severe or progressive clinical illness associated with suspected or confirmed influenza virus infection (i.e. clinical syndromes of pneumonia, sepsis or exacerbation of chronic underling diseases) should be treated with antiviral drug as soon as possible.

- Neuraminidase inhibitors (i.e. oseltamivir) should be prescribed as soon as possible (ideally, within 48 hours following symptom onset) to maximize therapeutic benefits. Administration of the drug should also be considered in patients presenting later in the course of illness.
- Treatment is recommended for a minimum of 5 days, but can be extended until there is satisfactory clinical improvement.

- Corticosteroids should not be used routinely, unless indicated for other reasons (eg: asthma and other specific conditions); as it has been associated with prolonged viral clearance, immunosuppression leading to bacterial or fungal superinfection.
- All currently circulating influenza viruses are resistant to adamantane antiviral drugs (such as amantadine and rimantadine), and these are therefore not recommended for monotherapy.[60]

The most effective way to prevent the disease is vaccination. Safe and effective vaccines are available and have been used for more than 60 years. Immunity from vaccination wanes over time so annual vaccination is recommended to protect against influenza. Injected inactivated influenza vaccines are most commonly used throughout the world.

Among healthy adults, influenza vaccine provides protection, even when circulating viruses do not exactly match the vaccine viruses. However, among the elderly, influenza vaccination may be less effective in preventing illness but reduces severity of disease and incidence of complications and deaths. Vaccination is especially important for people at high risk of influenza

[60] World Health Organization (2018), 'Influenza (Seasonal)', Available at: https://www.who.int/en/news-room/fact-sheets/detail/influenza-(seasonal) (accessed 2nd of August 2020).

complications, and for people who live with or care for the people at high risk.[61]

Apart from vaccination and antiviral treatment, the public health management includes personal protective measures like:

- Regular hand washing with proper drying of the hands
- Good respiratory hygiene – covering mouth and nose when coughing or sneezing, using tissues and disposing of them correctly
- Early self-isolation of those feeling unwell, feverish and having other symptoms of influenza
- Avoiding close contact with sick people
- Avoiding touching one's eyes, nose or mouth[62]

WHO, through the WHO GISRS system, in collaboration with other partners, monitors influenza activity globally, recommends seasonal influenza vaccine compositions twice a year for the Northern and Southern hemisphere influenza seasons, guides countries in tropical and subtropical areas to choose vaccine formulations (Northern hemisphere vs. Southern hemisphere), to support decisions for timing of vaccination

---

[61] World Health Organization (2018), 'Influenza (Seasonal)', Available at: https://www.who.int/en/news-room/fact-sheets/detail/influenza-(seasonal) (accessed 2nd of August 2020).

[62] World Health Organization (2018), 'Influenza (Seasonal)', Available at: https://www.who.int/en/news-room/fact-sheets/detail/influenza-(seasonal) (accessed 2nd of August 2020).

campaigns, and to support Member States to develop prevention and control strategies.[63]

1.1.8. PANDEMIC INFLUENZA

Pandemic influenza is an acute viral disease of the respiratory tract. It occurs when an influenza virus that was not previously circulating among people and to which most people have no immunity emerges and transmits among people.[64]

In June 2009, WHO declared the first influenza pandemic of the 21st century after the emergence of the new A(H1N1)pdm09 virus subtype. This virus was first isolated from humans in Mexico and the United States of America in April 2009. Within a few weeks, the virus had spread rapidly, and there was sustained human-to-human transmission worldwide. The triple-reassortant virus contained a unique combination of gene segments from avian, swine and human influenza viruses. Risk factors for severe influenza A(H1N1)pdm09 disease were similar to those for seasonal influenza, e.g. pregnancy and many chronic medical illnesses, although younger age groups were more affected than usual.

---

63 World Health Organization (2018), 'Influenza (Seasonal)', Available at: https://www.who.int/en/news-room/fact-sheets/detail/influenza-(seasonal) (accessed 2nd of August 2020).

64 World Health Organization (2020), 'Pandemic influenza: Introduction', Available at: https://openwho.org/courses/pandemic-influenza-introduction (accessed 3rd of August 2020).

Prior to 2009, much of the focus on influenza viruses with pandemic potential was on the avian influenza subtype A(H5N1). A human outbreak of avian influenza A(H5N1) was detected in 1997 in Hong Kong SAR, China. This was the first recognized instance in which a highly pathogenic avian influenza virus had been transmitted to humans and resulted in serious illness. Since its widespread re-emergence in 2003–2004, this avian virus has resulted in millions of poultry infections and over 800 human cases. On rare occasions, limited human-to-human transmission of influenza A(H5N1) has occurred – most often to a family or other household member acting as a caregiver. However, none of these events has so far resulted in sustained community-level transmission.[65]

Many animal influenza viruses naturally infect and circulate among a variety of avian and mammalian species. Most of these animal influenza viruses do not normally infect humans. However, on occasion, certain animal viruses do infect humans. Such infections have most often occurred as sporadic or isolated infections or sometimes resulted in small clusters of human infections. An influenza pandemic occurs when an animal influenza virus to which most humans have no immunity acquires the ability to cause sustained chains of human-to-

---

[65] World Health Organization. (2017). Pandemic influenza risk management: a WHO guide to inform and harmonize national and international pandemic preparedness and response. World Health Organization. https://apps.who.int/iris/handle/10665/259893. License: CC BY-NC-SA 3.0 IGO (accessed 2nd of August 2020).

human transmission leading to community-wide outbreaks. Such a virus has the potential to spread worldwide, causing a pandemic. The development of an influenza pandemic can be considered the result of the transformation of an animal influenza virus into a human influenza virus. At the genetic level, pandemic influenza viruses may arise through:

- genetic reassortment: a process in which genes from animal and human influenza viruses mix together to create a human-animal influenza reassortant virus;
- genetic mutation: a process in which genes in an animal influenza virus change allowing the virus to infect humans and transmit easily among them.[66]

Knowing who will do what, when, and with what resources is critical to managing a pandemic situation. Successful operations occur when actors know their roles and responsibilities, understand how they fit into the overall plan and how to work together, and have the capacities and resources to implement the plan. To achieve these objectives, all stakeholders need to be involved in the planning process – the process is as important as the plan itself.[67]

---

[66] World Health Organization (2009), 'PANDEMIC INFLUENZA PREPAREDNESS AND RESPONSE', Available at: https://www.who.int/influenza/resources/documents/pandemic_guidance_04_2009/en/ (accessed 3rd of August 2020).

[67] World Health Organization (2018), 'A checklist for pandemic influenza risk and impact management: building capacity for pandemic response', Available at:

1.1.9. HUMAN IMMUNODEFICIENCY VIRUS (HIV)

HIV (human immunodeficiency virus) is a virus that attacks the body's immune system. If HIV is not treated, it can lead to AIDS (acquired immunodeficiency syndrome).[68] You can get or transmit HIV only through specific activities. Most commonly, people get or transmit HIV through sexual behaviors and needle or syringe use. Only certain body fluids—blood, semen (cum), pre-seminal fluid (pre-cum), rectal fluids, vaginal fluids, and breast milk—from a person who has HIV can transmit HIV. These fluids must come in contact with a mucous membrane or damaged tissue or be directly injected into the bloodstream (from a needle or syringe) for transmission to occur. Mucous membranes are found inside the rectum, vagina, penis, and mouth.[69]

Today, more tools than ever are available to prevent HIV. You can use strategies such as abstinence (not having sex), limiting your number of sexual partners, never sharing needles, and using condoms the right way every time you have sex. You may also be able to take advantage of newer HIV prevention

---

https://www.who.int/influenza/preparedness/pandemic/influenza_risk_management_checklist_2018/en/ (accessed 3rd of August 2020).

[68] United States Centers for Disease Control and Prevention (2020), 'About HIV', Available at: https://www.cdc.gov/hiv/basics/whatishiv.html (accessed 26 July 2020).

[69] United States Centers for Disease Control and Prevention (2019), 'HIV Transmission', Available at: https://www.cdc.gov/hiv/basics/transmission.html (accessed 26 July 2020).

medicines such as pre-exposure prophylaxis (PrEP) and post-exposure prophylaxis (PEP).

If you have HIV, there are many actions you can take to prevent transmitting it to others. The most important is taking HIV medicine (called antiretroviral therapy, or ART) as prescribed. If you take HIV medicine as prescribed and get and keep an undetectable viral load (or stay virally suppressed), you can stay healthy and have effectively no risk of transmitting HIV to an HIV-negative sex partner.[70]

1.2. THE GLOBAL APPROACH TO COMBATING INFECTIOUS DISEASES

New challenges to human health require new strategies for evaluating and managing EID risks as part of the International Health Regulations (IHR 2005) monitoring and evaluation framework.[71] Successful implementation of IHR 2005 requires the fulfilment of 8 core capacities: legislation, policy and

---

[70] United States Centers for Disease Control and Prevention (2019), 'Prevention', Available at: https://www.cdc.gov/hiv/basics/prevention.html (accessed 26 July 2020).

[71] The International Health Regulations (IHR) is a set of regulations adopted by 194 WHO Member States to govern surveillance of public health emergencies of international concern. They were enacted in 2005 and came into force on 15 June 2007 and are legally binding for WHO Member States. In 2006, the Resolution AFR/RC56/R2 of the Regional Committee for Africa in Addis Ababa called for the implementation of the IHR (2005) in the context of Integrated Disease Surveillance and Response (IDSR).

coordination, surveillance, preparedness, response, risk communications, laboratory and human resources.[72]

A range of response planning strategies has been developed to attempt to identify new infectious threats as they emerge to facilitate a timely response, including control. This chapter will expound on these strategies with a focus on the World Health Organization, the United States' Centers for Disease Control and Prevention, the United Kingdom's Department of Health and the Nigeria Centre for Disease Control.

1.2.1. THE WORLD HEALTH ORGANIZATION

The World Health Organization (WHO) is responsible for providing leadership on global health matters, shaping the health research agenda, setting norms and standards, articulating evidence-based policy options, providing technical support to Member States, and monitoring and assessing health trends. WHO promotes health as a shared responsibility, involving equitable access to essential care and collective defence against transnational threats.[73]

In 2009, WHO used six phases of pandemic alert as a system for informing the world of the seriousness of the threat. These

[72] International Health Regulations 2005, Annex 1.

[73] World Health Organization (2017), 'Pandemic Influenza Risk Management Guidance', Available at: https://www.who.int/influenza/preparedness/pandemic/influenza_risk_management_update2017/en/ (accessed 1st of August 2020).

phases reflect the progression of an influenza pandemic from the first appearance of a new flu virus to wide international spread.[74]

In Phase 1 no viruses circulating among animals have been reported to cause infections in humans.

In Phase 2 an animal influenza virus circulating among domesticated or wild animals is known to have caused infection in humans, and is therefore considered a potential pandemic threat.

In Phase 3, an animal or human-animal influenza reassortant virus has caused sporadic cases or small clusters of disease in people, but has not resulted in human-to-human transmission sufficient to sustain community-level outbreaks. Limited human-to-human transmission may occur under some circumstances, for example, when there is close contact between an infected person and an unprotected caregiver. However, limited transmission under such restricted circumstances does not indicate that the virus has gained the level of transmissibility among humans necessary to cause a pandemic.

Phase 4 is characterized by verified human-to-human transmission of an animal or human-animal influenza reassortant virus able to cause "community-level outbreaks." The

---

[74] Ireland's Health Service Executive (HSE) together with the Department of Health and Children (2007), 'National Pandemic Influenza Plan', Available at: https://www.gov.ie/en/publication/d9ce58-national-pandemic-influenza-plan/?referrer=http://www.health.gov.ie/blog/publications/national-pandemic-influenza-plan (accessed 29 July 2020).

ability to cause sustained disease outbreaks in a community marks a significant upwards shift in the risk for a pandemic. Any country that suspects or has verified such an event should urgently consult with WHO so that the situation can be jointly assessed, and a decision made by the affected country if implementation of a rapid pandemic containment operation is warranted. Phase 4 indicates a significant increase in risk of a pandemic but does not necessarily mean that a pandemic is a forgone conclusion.

Phase 5 is characterized by human-to-human spread of the virus into at least two countries in one WHO region. While most countries will not be affected at this stage, the declaration of Phase 5 is a strong signal that a pandemic is imminent and that the time to finalize the organization, communication, and implementation of the planned mitigation measures is short.

Phase 6, the pandemic phase, is characterized by community level outbreaks in at least one other country in a different WHO region in addition to the criteria defined in Phase 5. Designation of this phase will indicate that a global pandemic is under way.[75]

In 2017, WHO updated its previous pandemic preparedness guidance and checklist with lessons learned from the 2009 influenza pandemic, introduced the strategies and approaches in

---

[75] World Health Organization (2009), 'Emergencies preparedness, response: Current WHO phase of pandemic alert for Pandemic (H1N1) 2009', Available at: https://www.who.int/csr/disease/swineflu/phase/en/ (accessed 1st of August 2020).

pandemic influenza risk and impact management, and emphasized the importance of national risk and severity assessments in guiding the national response actions.

Currently, there are four WHO global pandemic phases:

- ***interpandemic*** – the period between influenza pandemics;
- ***alert*** – influenza caused by a new subtype has been identified in humans; therefore, increased vigilance and careful risk assessment will be initiated at local, national and global levels;
- ***pandemic***– global spread of human influenza caused by a new subtype, determined through global surveillance; and
- ***transition*** – reduction of assessed global risk, de-escalation of global actions and reduction in response activities or movement towards recovery.

The designation of alert phases, including decisions on when to move from one phase to another, is made by the Director-General of the World Health Organization. The transition between phases may be rapid and some phases may be skipped. Each alert phase coincides with a series of recommended activities to be undertaken by WHO, the international community, Governments and industry. Changes from one phase to another are triggered by several factors, which include the behaviour of the disease and the characteristics of circulating viruses.[76]

1.2.2. UNITED STATES CENTERS FOR DISEASE CONTROL AND PREVENTION

Centers for Disease Control and Prevention (CDC) is the United States leading science-based, data-driven, service organization that protects the public's health. For more than 70 years, the CDC put science into action to help children stay healthy so they can grow and learn, to help families, businesses and communities respond to and prevent disease outbreaks and stay strong, and to protect the public's health.[77]

CDC's Strategic Framework & Priorities to save American lives cascade from an ambitious aspiration, into granular action plans, and detailed measures of success. The Strategic Framework & Priorities were built with the input of about 100 of CDC's experts, and reflects both the Director's decades of research in virology, infectious diseases, and epidemiology, along

---

[76] World Health Organization (2017), 'Pandemic Influenza Risk Management Guidance', Available at: https://www.who.int/influenza/preparedness/pandemic/influenza_risk_management_update2017/en/ (accessed 1st of August 2020).

[77] United States Centers for Disease Control and Prevention (2020), 'A Bold Promise to the Nation', Available at: https://www.cdc.gov/about/24-7/index.html (accessed 2nd of August 2020).

with CDC's deep knowledge and many years of experience responding to and preventing disease outbreaks.[78]

In 2011, the United States' Centers for Disease Control and Prevention (CDC) established 15 capabilities that serve as national standards for public health preparedness planning.[79] The United States Healthcare Preparedness Capabilities planning model is based on a planning process that healthcare systems, healthcare coalitions and healthcare organization may wish to utilize to help determine their preparedness priorities and plan their preparedness activities. This process fits into the planning phase of the U.S. Department of Homeland Security (DHS) preparedness cycle and is outlined in Chapter 4 of the DHS Federal Emergency Management Agency's Developing and Maintaining Emergency Operations Plans, Comprehensive Preparedness Guide (CPG) 101, Version 2.0.[80]

---

[78] United States Centers for Disease Control and Prevention (2019), 'CDC's Strategic Framework & Priorities: 2019 Progress Report', Available at: https://www.cdc.gov/about/pdf/StrategicPrioritiesReport.pdf (accessed 2nd of August 2020).

[79] United States Centers for Disease Control and Prevention (2011), 'Public Health Preparedness Capabilities: National Standards for State and Local Planning', Available at: https://idph.iowa.gov/Portals/1/userfiles/61/Preparedness/PHEP%20Preparedness%20Capabilities_March_2011.pdf (accessed 24 July 2020).

[80] United States Department of Health and Human Services, Office of the Assistant Secretary for Preparedness and Response (2012), 'Healthcare Preparedness Capabilities: National Guidance for Healthcare System Preparedness: January 2012', Available at: http://www.phe.gov/preparedness/planning/hpp/reports/documents/capabilities.pdf (accessed 25 July 2020).

Over the years, feedback from subject matter experts (SMEs) across CDC, state and local health departments, and national partner organizations highlighted specific opportunities to revise and modernize the capabilities. In 2017, CDC began updating the capabilities in response to lessons learned from public health emergency responses, updates to public health preparedness science, revised guidance and resources, findings from internal reviews and assessments, SME feedback from the practice community, and input from allied federal agencies. In addition, representatives from professional associations, including the Association of Public Health Laboratories (APHL), the Association of State and Territorial Health Officials (ASTHO), the Council of State and Territorial Epidemiologists (CSTE), the National Association of County and City Health Officials (NACCHO), and the National Emergency Management Association (NEMA) provided input on the updated content.[81]

The capabilities update focused on streamlining language and aligning content with new national standards, updated science, and current public health priorities and strategies. The capabilities also support topics such as pandemic influenza,

[81] United States Centers for Disease Control and Prevention (2018), 'Public Health Emergency Preparedness and Response Capabilities: National Standards for State, Local, Tribal, and Territorial Public Health', Available at: https://www.cdc.gov/cpr/readiness/capabilities.htm (accessed 24 July 2020).

environmental health, at-risk populations, and tribal populations.[82]

The 2018 Public Health Emergency Preparedness and Response Capabilities: National Standards for State, Local, Tribal, and Territorial Public Health recognizes the maturity and experience jurisdictional public health emergency preparedness and response programs have gained since 2011. The document describes the components necessary to advance jurisdictional public health preparedness and response capacity.

PHASE 1: ASSESS CURRENT STATE

The first step in the assessment phase is to determine which organizational entities within the jurisdiction are responsible for each domain, capability standard, and applicable capability resource elements. Organizational entities may include allied state agencies, such as emergency management, partner organizations, other jurisdictional public health agencies, health care coalitions, community-based partners, and other jurisdictional stakeholders.

---

[82] United States Centers for Disease Control and Prevention (2018), 'Public Health Emergency Preparedness and Response Capabilities: National Standards for State, Local, Tribal, and Territorial Public Health', Available at: https://www.cdc.gov/cpr/readiness/capabilities.htm (accessed 24 July 2020).

PHASE 2: DETERMINE STRATEGIES AND ACTIVITIES

In addition to assessing and reviewing capability resource elements, jurisdictions should review supplementary information sources to help identify jurisdictional needs and gaps. Supplementary information sources may include

- Existing data from jurisdictional hazard vulnerability analyses (jurisdictional risk assessment findings)
- Jurisdictional intelligence data, such as fusion center data or information obtained from intelligence reports or briefings
- Jurisdictional emergency management response plans, such as scenario-based plans
- Funding considerations, such as guidance or funding requirements from related federal preparedness programs
- Current public health strategic plans or strategic priorities
- Previous state and local accreditation or recognition efforts, such as Project Public Health Ready and Public Health Accreditation Board standards
- Jurisdictional results or action plans resulting from CDC operational readiness reviews
- After-action reports and corrective action plans

Phase 3: Develop Plans

Jurisdictional public health agencies should establish concrete organizational initiatives and plan activities to achieve short- and long-term goals. For the purposes of this planning model, an assumption is made that activities specifically relate to individual capability domains, capability definitions, capability functions, capability tasks, and capability resource elements. However, in practice, jurisdictional public health agencies may group related activities to address multiple capability standards within any single project or program development initiative.[83]

1.2.3. UNITED KINGDOM'S DEPARTMENT OF HEALTH

Influenza pandemic planning in the UK has been based on an assessment of the "reasonable worst case". This is derived from the experience and a mathematical analysis of influenza pandemics and seasonal influenza in the 20th century. This suggests that, given known patterns of spread of infection, up to 50 per cent of the population could experience symptoms of pandemic influenza during one or more pandemic waves lasting

[83] United States Centers for Disease Control and Prevention (2018), 'Public Health Emergency Preparedness and Response Capabilities: National Standards for State, Local, Tribal, and Territorial Public Health', Available at: https://www.cdc.gov/cpr/readiness/00_docs/CDC_PreparednesResponseCapabilities_October2018_Final_508.pdf (accessed 24 July 2020).

15 weeks, although the nature and severity of the symptoms would vary from person to person.[84]

The United Kingdom has developed a new approach to the indicators for action in a future pandemic response. This takes the form of a series of phases, named: Detection, Assessment, Treatment, Escalation and Recovery and incorporates indicators for moving from one phase to another.

Detection – This phase would commence on either the declaration of the current WHO phase 2 (formerly phase 4) or earlier on the basis of reliable intelligence that there is verified human-to-human transmission of an animal or human-animal influenza reassortant virus able to cause "community-level outbreaks or if an influenza-related "Public Health Emergency of International Concern" (a "PHEIC") is declared by the WHO. The focus in this stage would be:

- Intelligence gathering from countries already affected.
- Enhanced surveillance within the UK.
- The development of diagnostics specific to the new virus.

[84] United Kingdom's Department of Health (2011), 'UK Influenza Pandemic Preparedness Strategy', Available at: https://www.gov.uk/government/publications/review-of-the-evidence-base-underpinning-the-uk-influenza-pandemic-preparedness-strategy (accessed 29 July 2020).

- Information and communications to the public and professionals.

The indicator for moving to the next stage would be the identification of the novel influenza virus in patients in the UK.[85]

Assessment – The focus in this stage would be:

- The collection and analysis of detailed clinical and epidemiological information on early cases, on which to base early estimates of impact and severity in the UK.
- Reducing the risk of transmission and infection with the virus within the local community by:
    - - actively finding cases;
    - - self isolation of cases and suspected cases; and
    - - treatment of cases / suspected cases and use of antiviral prophylaxis for close / vulnerable contacts, based on a risk assessment of the possible impact of the disease.

---

85 United Kingdom's Department of Health (2011), 'UK Influenza Pandemic Preparedness Strategy', Available at: https://www.gov.uk/government/publications/review-of-the-evidence-base-underpinning-the-uk-influenza-pandemic-preparedness-strategy (accessed 29 July 2020).

The indicator for moving from this stage would be evidence of sustained community transmission of the virus, i.e. cases not linked to any known or previously identified cases.

These two stages – Detection and Assessment - together form the initial response. This may be relatively short and the phases may be combined depending on the speed with which the virus spreads, or the severity with which individuals and communities are affected. It will not be possible to halt the spread of a new pandemic influenza virus, and it would be a waste of public health resources and capacity to attempt to do so.[86]

Treatment – The focus in this stage would be:

- Treatment of individual cases and population treatment via the National Pandemic Flu Service (NPFS), if necessary.
- Enhancement of the health response to deal with increasing numbers of cases.
- Consider enhancing public health measures to disrupt local transmission of the virus as appropriate, such as localised school closures based on public health risk assessment.

---

[86] United Kingdom's Department of Health (2011), 'UK Influenza Pandemic Preparedness Strategy', Available at: https://www.gov.uk/government/publications/review-of-the-evidence-base-underpinning-the-uk-influenza-pandemic-preparedness-strategy (accessed 29 July 2020).

- Depending upon the development of the pandemic, to prepare for targeted vaccinations as the vaccine becomes available.

Arrangements will be activated to ensure that necessary detailed surveillance activity continues in relation to samples of community cases, hospitalised cases and deaths.

When demands for services start to exceed the available capacity, additional measures will need to be taken. This decision is likely to be made at a regional or local level as not all parts of the UK will be affected at the same time or to the same degree of intensity.[87]

Escalation – The focus in this stage would be:

- Escalation of surge management arrangements in health and other sectors.
- Prioritisation and triage of service delivery with aim to maintain essential services.
- Resiliency measures, encompassing robust contingency plans.
- Consideration of de-escalation of response if the situation is judged to have improved sufficiently.

---

[87] United Kingdom's Department of Health (2011), 'UK Influenza Pandemic Preparedness Strategy 2011', Available at: https://www.gov.uk/government/publications/review-of-the-evidence-base-underpinning-the-uk-influenza-pandemic-preparedness-strategy (accessed 29 July 2020).

These two stages form the Treatment phase of the pandemic. Whilst escalation measures may not be needed in mild pandemics, it would be prudent to prepare for the implementation of the Escalation phase at an early stage of the Treatment phase, if not before.[88]

Recovery – The focus in this stage would be:

- Normalisation of services, perhaps to a new definition of what constitutes normal service.
- Restoration of business as usual services, including an element of catching-up with activity that may have been scaled-down as part of the pandemic response e.g. reschedule routine operations.
- Post-incident review of response, and sharing information on what went well, what could be improved, and lessons learnt.
- Taking steps to address staff exhaustion.
- Planning and preparation for a resurgence of influenza, including activities carried out in the Detection phase.
- Continuing to consider targeted vaccination, when available.

---

[88] United Kingdom's Department of Health (2011), 'UK Influenza Pandemic Preparedness Strategy 2011', Available at: https://www.gov.uk/government/publications/review-of-the-evidence-base-underpinning-the-uk-influenza-pandemic-preparedness-strategy (accessed 29 July 2020).

- Preparing for post-pandemic seasonal influenza.

The indicator for this phase would be when influenza activity is either significantly reduced compared to the peak or when the activity is considered to be within acceptable parameters. An overview of how services' capacities are able to meet demand will also inform this decision.[89]

1.2.4. NIGERIA CENTRE FOR DISEASE CONTROL

The Nigeria Centre for Disease Control (NCDC) was established in the year 2011 in response to the challenges of public health emergencies and to enhance Nigeria's preparedness and response to epidemics through prevention, detection and control of communicable diseases.[90] Its core mandate is to detect, investigate, prevent and control diseases of national and international public health importance. The mission for the NCDC next five years (2017-2021) is 'to protect the health of Nigerians through evidence-based prevention, integrated disease surveillance and response activities, using a One Health

89 United Kingdom's Department of Health (2011), 'UK Influenza Pandemic Preparedness Strategy 2011', Available at: https://www.gov.uk/government/publications/review-of-the-evidence-base-underpinning-the-uk-influenza-pandemic-preparedness-strategy (accessed 29 July 2020).

90 Nigeria Centre for Disease Control (2020), 'Mandate of NCDC', Available at: https://ncdc.gov.ng/ (accessed 4 September 2020).

approach, guided by research and led by a skilled workforce.' The core functions of the NCDC include:

- **Prevent, detect, and control** diseases of public health importance
- **Coordinate** surveillance systems to collect, analyse and interpret data on diseases of public health importance
- **Support** States in responding to small outbreaks and lead the response to large disease outbreaks
- **Develop** and maintain a network of reference and specialsed laboratories
- **Lead Nigeria's engagement** with the international community on diseases of public health relevance
- **Conduct, collate, synthesize and disseminate** public health research to inform policy[91]

Over the past 4 years, Nigeria has been confronted with several outbreaks of epidemic-prone diseases, including measles, yellow fever, cerebrospinal meningitis, cholera, Lassa fever, and monkeypox. In response to some of these disease outbreaks, public health workers have conducted vaccination campaigns, while also providing infection prevention and control training to

---

[91] Federal Ministry of Health, Federal Ministry of Agriculture and Rural Development and Federal Ministry of Environment (2019), 'One Health Strategic Plan 2019–2023', Available at: https://ncdc.gov.ng/themes/common/docs/protocols/93_1566785462.pdf (accessed 4 September 2020).

health workers, establishing new laboratory testing capacity, and conducting communication and engagement activities to communities. The Nigeria Centre for Disease Control (NCDC), which serves as the National Focal Point for the International Health Regulations (2005) (IHR NFP), is responsible for surveillance and response to these outbreaks, and works closely with the National Primary Healthcare Development Agency (NPHCDA) when a vaccination response is needed.[92]

[92] The Government of Nigeria (2018), 'National Action Plan for Health Security Federal Republic of Nigeria (2018-2022)', Available at: https://ncdc.gov.ng/themes/common/files/establishment/5e88f9e22d2b4e4563b527005c8a0c43.pdf (accessed 27 August 2020).

CHAPTER 2

OVERVIEW OF THE METHODOLOGY TO ASSESS PUBLIC HEALTH RISKS AND EVENTS AT THE NATIONAL LEVEL

Risk can be defined as the likelihood of an event and its consequences. In simple terms, risk can be seen as a combination of the chance that something may happen and the degree of damage or loss that may result from such an occurrence.[93]

Risk assessment is a systematic process for gathering, assessing and documenting information to assign a level of risk. It provides the basis for taking action to manage and reduce the negative consequences of acute public health risks.[94] Risk assessment is an integral part of the wider process of risk analysis, which starts with hazard identification, and includes risk

[93] Financial Transactions and Reporting Analysis Centre of Canada: Guidance on the Risk-Based Approach to Combatting Money laundering and Terrorist Financing 2015, page 4.

[94] World Health Organization (2012), 'Rapid Risk Assessment of Acute Public Health Events', Available at: https://www.who.int/csr/resources/publications/HSE_GAR_ARO_2012_1/en/ (accessed 4th of June 2020).

management and communication.[95] The risk management cycle includes:

- **risk assessment** — The level of risk assigned to an event is based on the suspected (or known) hazard, the possible exposure to the hazard, and the context in which the event is occurring. Risk assessment includes three components — hazard, exposure, and context assessments. The outcome of these three assessments is used to characterize the overall level of risk.[96] In hazard identification, an association between disease and the presence of a pathogen in a food is documented. The information may describe conditions under which the pathogen survives, grows, causes infection, and dies. Epidemiologic and surveillance data, challenge testing, and scientific studies of pathogenicity also contribute information. Data collected during hazard identification are later used in exposure assessment, where the impact of processing, distribution, preparation, and consumption of the food are incorporated.[97]

[95] Morgan D, Kirkbride H, Hewitt K, Said B, Walsh AL. Assessing the risk from emerging infections. *Epidemiol Infect.* 2009;137(11):1521-1530. doi:10.1017/S0950268809990227 (accessed 4th of June 2020).

[96] World Health Organization (2012), 'Rapid Risk Assessment of Acute Public Health Events', Available at: https://www.who.int/csr/resources/publications/HSE_GAR_ARO_2012_1/en/ (accessed 4th of June 2020).

[97] Lammerding, A. M., & Paoli, G. M. (1997). Quantitative risk assessment: an emerging tool for emerging foodborne pathogens. *Emerging infectious diseases, 3*(4), 483–487. https://doi.org/10.3201/eid0304.970411 (accessed 4th of June 2020).

Exposure assessment describes the pathways through which a pathogen population is introduced, distributed, and challenged in the production, distribution, and consumption of food. This step differs from hazard identification in that it describes a particular food-processing pathway. Dose-response assessment is used to translate the final exposure to a pathogen population into a health response in the population of consumers.[98]

- **identification of potential control measures** — The outcome of a risk assessment should be used to direct proportionate control measures that reflect the risk. The overall level of risk assigned to the event helps identify the urgency and extent of the control measures needed. Both risk matrices can also be used to rank control measures according to their effectiveness. For example, they can be used to rank the likelihood that a control measure will prevent further spread or dissemination of a hazard and the consequences of applying each control measure.[99]
- **monitoring and evaluation** – A risk assessment should be repeated as new information becomes

[98] Lammerding, A. M., & Paoli, G. M. (1997). Quantitative risk assessment: an emerging tool for emerging foodborne pathogens. *Emerging infectious diseases*, *3*(4), 483–487. https://doi.org/10.3201/eid0304.970411 (accessed 6th of June 2020).
[99] World Health Organization (2012), 'Rapid Risk Assessment of Acute Public Health Events', Available at: https://www.who.int/csr/resources/publications/HSE_GAR_ARO_2012_1/en/ (accessed 4th of June 2020).

available. It may also be repeated on a regular timetable (e.g. daily in the early stages of an event, perhaps driven by a Minister who agrees to provide an update to other Ministers or to the media at a specific time each day).[100]

A common approach to risk assessment is the amalgamation of a range of objective and subjective data to produce risk-related standards. Events which are on-going, unfolding or 'one off' must be considered in the assessment of a specific threat. Many of these techniques can be adapted and applied to public health, where it is particularly important to recognize the potentially significant consequences of seemingly small risks.[101] At the outset of a potential epidemic, a priority is to assess whether the new disease will spread on a sustained basis—the assessment of transmissibility.[102] A prominent example, central to our current understanding of epidemic spread, is the basic reproductive number, (R_0), which is defined as the mean number of infections caused by an infected individual in a susceptible population. Population estimates of (R_0) can obscure considerable individual

---

100 World Health Organization (2012), 'Rapid Risk Assessment of Acute Public Health Events', Available at: https://www.who.int/csr/resources/publications/HSE_GAR_ARO_2012_1/en/ (accessed 4th of June 2020).

101 Morgan D, Kirkbride H, Hewitt K, Said B, Walsh AL. Assessing the risk from emerging infections. *Epidemiol Infect.* 2009;137(11):1521-1530. doi:10.1017/S0950268809990227 (accessed 6th of June 2020).

102 David N Fisman, Gabriel M Leung and Marc Lipsitch (2014), 'Nuanced risk assessment for emerging infectious diseases', The Lancet, VOLUME 383, ISSUE 9913, P189-190, https://www.thelancet.com/journals/lancet/article/PIIS0140-6736(13)62123-6/fulltext (accessed 7th of June 2020).

variation in infectiousness, as highlighted during the global emergence of severe acute respiratory syndrome (SARS) by numerous 'superspreading events' in which certain individuals infected unusually large numbers of secondary cases.[103]

The **International Health Regulations (IHR) 2005** provide the legal framework for the timely and effective management of a broad range of serious and potentially international public health risks and events. In addition, the Regulations provide a specialized mechanism for collective global action for certain rare events of particular importance. Such serious events that endanger global public health are specified by the Regulations as a Public Health Emergency of International Concern (PHEIC).[104] The term is defined in the IHR (2005) as "an extraordinary event which is determined to constitute a public health risk to other States through the international spread of disease and to potentially require a coordinated international response". This definition implies a situation that: is serious, unusual or unexpected; carries implications for public health beyond the affected State's national border; and may require coordinated international action.[105]

---

[103] Lloyd-Smith, J. O., Schreiber, S. J., Kopp, P. E. & Getz, W. M. (2005), 'Superspreading and the effect of individual variation on disease emergence', Vol 438|17, https://www.nature.com/articles/nature04153.pdf (accessed 7th of June 2020).

[104] International Health Regulations 2005, Article 6.

[105] International Health Regulations 2005, Article 1.

The responsibility of determining whether an event is within this category lies with the World Health Organization (WHO) Director-General[106] and requires the convening of a committee of health experts – the IHR Emergency Committee.[107] This Committee advises the Director-General on recommended measures to be implemented on an emergency basis, known as temporary recommendations. Temporary recommendations may include health measures to be implemented by the State Party experiencing the PHEIC, or by other States Parties, to prevent or reduce the international spread of disease and avoid unnecessary interference with international traffic.[108]

The IHR (2005) also provide a mandate to WHO to perform public health surveillance, risk assessment, support States Parties, and coordinate the international response to significant international public health risks and events.[109] After preliminary assessment, WHO is obliged by the IHR (2005) to obtain verification from States Parties of unofficial reports of events that may constitute a PHEIC.[110] If verification is sought, including in the context of potential pandemic influenza, States Parties are required to respond to WHO within a prescribed time period and include available relevant public health information.[111] The legal requirement to respond to requests for

---

106 International Health Regulations 2005, Article 12(1).
107 International Health Regulations 2005, Article 12(2).
108 International Health Regulations 2005, Article 15.
109 International Health Regulations 2005, Article 5(3) and Article 5(4).
110 International Health Regulations 2005, Article 10(1).
111 International Health Regulations 2005, Article 10(2).

verification by WHO aims to provide early identification and assessment of, and response to, any public health event with international implications.[112] WHO is also obligated to provide public health information to all States Parties as soon as possible regarding public health risks, to enable them to respond and protect their populations. When WHO intends to make information available to other States Parties, it has an obligation to consult with the country experiencing the event.[113]

In line with the mandate given to it by IHR (2005), WHO has published several key documents to support global pandemic preparedness efforts. In 2017 and early 2018, WHO published several key documents to support global pandemic preparedness efforts. The pandemic influenza risk management (PIRM) document and its supporting checklist update the previous WHO pandemic preparedness guidance and checklist with lessons learned from the 2009 influenza pandemic, introduce the strategies and approaches in pandemic influenza risk and impact management, and emphasize the importance of national risk and severity assessments in guiding the national response actions. The *WHO simulation exercise manual* provides guidance on the concepts and principles for conducting and managing

---

112 World Health Organization (2017), 'Pandemic Influenza Risk Management Guidance', Available at: https://apps.who.int/iris/bitstream/handle/10665/259893/WHO-WHE-IHM-GIP-2017.1-eng.pdf;jsessionid=8C9EFCECED9F0B80A01F4B4642683941?sequence=1 (accessed 1st of August 2020).

113 International Health Regulations 2005, Article 11.

simulation exercises. This current guide introduces a risk-based approach to pandemic influenza risk management and encourages Member States to develop flexible plans based on national risk assessment, taking account of the global risk assessment conducted by WHO.

It is worth noting that countries around the world have developed flexible set of measures, through a rigorous and systematic analysis of qualitative and quantitative data and expert opinion about threats and hazards of concern. This chapter provides an overview of the national risk assessment methodology with a focus on the United States of America, the United Kingdom and Nigeria.

2.1. UNITED STATES

The 2019 National Threat and Hazard Identification and Risk Assessment (National THIRA) represents an initial effort to identify the greatest threats and hazards to the United States of America, the potential impacts of those threats and hazards to life and property, and the capabilities needed to address those impacts. Since 2012, communities have used a standard THIRA methodology to identify and assess the threats and hazards they face. In 2018, this methodology was updated to include new standardized language. The National THIRA applies the updated THIRA methodology and the standardized language at the national level to answer the following key questions:

- Which realistic threats and hazards will be the most challenging for the Nation to manage?
- If they occurred, what impacts would those threats and hazards have on the Nation?
- Based on those impacts, what capabilities will the Nation need to manage the incident?

The National THIRA describes the level of capability that the Nation—including government, private, and non-profit sectors—would need to fully manage the Nation's threats and hazards of greatest concern while concurrently engaging in response and recovery efforts for ongoing disasters.

The following section provides an overview of the three-step methodology Federal Emergency Management Agency's (FEMA) used to develop the 2019 National THIRA. The THIRA process that FEMA used is consistent with the Comprehensive Preparedness Guide (CPG) 201, 3rd Edition, applied at the national level.[114]

2.1.1. Identify Threats and Hazards of Concern

[114] United States Federal Emergency Management Agency (2019), '2019 National Threat and Hazard Identification and Risk Assessment (THIRA): Overview and Methodology', Available at: https://www.fema.gov/sites/default/files/2020-06/fema_national-thira-overview-methodology_2019_0.pdf (accessed 24 August 2020).

FEMA considered two factors when evaluating which threats and hazards to include in the National THIRA: 1) whether the threat or hazard could realistically affect the Nation; and 2) the challenge the threat or hazard would present to the Nation's capabilities if it occurred. FEMA ultimately included nine scenarios spread across six threats and hazards that could realistically occur and challenge the Nation's capabilities. By having a uniform, prioritized list of the Nation's realistic worst-case scenarios, Federal agencies and other partner organizations involved in incident management will be better able to coordinate their planning and exercises efforts.

FEMA developed a research agenda and refined the threat and hazard list in four steps:

1. Conducted a literature review to develop a preliminary list of threats and hazards.
2. Consulted with subject-matter experts (SMEs) to identify the most challenging threats and hazards to the core capabilities.
3. Solicited stakeholder feedback to refine most challenging threats and hazards, and
4. Refined the threat and hazard list based on available data and SME review.[115]

[115] United States Federal Emergency Management Agency (2019), '2019 National Threat and Hazard Identification

2.1.2. Give Threats and Hazards Context

Context descriptions allow FEMA to determine why certain threats and hazards are particularly challenging for the Nation to address. They also provide key information that helps FEMA measure the estimated impacts of threats and hazards.

Through Step 2 of the National THIRA, FEMA developed context descriptions for each of the threats and hazards identified in Step 1. Context descriptions, framed as narratives of potential scenarios, indicate what factors would make each threat or hazard especially challenging for the Nation, including location, magnitude, time of an incident, and cascading effects. In Step 2, FEMA also estimated the potential impacts of each scenario.[116]

2.1.3. Establish Capability Targets

Capability targets include specific and measurable metrics that describe the capabilities the Nation needs to manage potential catastrophic incidents. Additionally, the capability targets establish a benchmark that the emergency management community can use to track progress over time, allowing the

---

and Risk Assessment (THIRA): Overview and Methodology', Available at: https://www.fema.gov/sites/default/files/2020-06/fema_national-thira-overview-methodology_2019_0.pdf (accessed 24 August 2020).

[116] United States Federal Emergency Management Agency (2019), '2019 National Threat and Hazard Identification
and Risk Assessment (THIRA): Overview and Methodology', Available at: https://www.fema.gov/sites/default/files/2020-06/fema_national-thira-overview-methodology_2019_0.pdf (accessed 24 August 2020).

Nation to assess how it currently responds to threats and hazards, as well as how it can improve.

For Step 3 of the National THIRA process, FEMA created standard language, that when combined with scenario impact data and operational timeframe metrics, became national capability targets. These targets are specific benchmarks for measuring how prepared the Nation is for the potential impacts of its most challenging threats and hazards.

FEMA developed 22 standardized targets for the 2019 National THIRA. The standardized targets represent a common set of measures that communities use to conduct a more comprehensive, unified assessment across all levels of emergency management. The targets in this report demonstrate the massive response and recovery efforts that would be needed to address the catastrophic-level impacts of potential disasters. National targets will allow the emergency management community and all levels of government to better synchronize preparedness efforts and plan for these disasters.[117]

Although the three-step methodology FEMA used to develop the 2019 National THIRA was able to successfully identify the greatest threats and hazards to the United States

117 United States Federal Emergency Management Agency (2019), '2019 National Threat and Hazard Identification and Risk Assessment (THIRA): Overview and Methodology', Available at: https://www.fema.gov/sites/default/files/2020-06/fema_national-thira-overview-methodology_2019_0.pdf (accessed 24 August 2020).

of America, there is little that is specific to the assessment of emerging public health threats at the national level.

2.2 UNITED KINGDOM

Since 2005, the Government of the United Kingdom (UK) has carried out a classified assessment of the risks facing the United Kingdom: this is the National Risk Assessment (NRA), and it is the basis for the public National Risk Register. The NRA process uses historical and scientific data, and the professional judgements of experts to analyse the risks to the UK. There are three stages to this analysis: identification of risks; assessment of the likelihood of the risks occurring and their impact if they do; and comparison of the risks.[118]

2.2.1. Identifying risks

The first stage in the National Risk Assessment process is to identify the risks. This is done by consulting a wide range of experts across government, so as to ensure a comprehensive picture of the potential accidents, natural events (hazards) and malicious attacks (threats) that could cause significant harm and disruption to the UK.[119]

---

118 United Kingdom's Cabinet Office (2008), 'National Risk Register', Available at: https://assets.publishing.service.gov.uk/government/uploads/system/uploads/attachment_data/file/61934/national_risk_register.pdf (accessed 24 August 2020).

119 United Kingdom's Cabinet Office (2008), 'National Risk Register', Available at: https://assets.publishing.service.gov.uk/government/uploads/system/uploads/attachment_data/file/61934/national_risk_register.pdf (accessed 24 August 2020).

2.2.2. Assessing risks

The next stage is to assess the likelihood and impact of each risk. To assess the likelihood of hazards, historical, statistical and scientific data are used. Where possible, the assessment looks forward to take account of known or probable developments over the next five years that would affect the likelihood.

The likelihood of terrorist or other malicious attacks is assessed more subjectively. The willingness of individuals or groups to carry out attacks is balanced against an objective assessment of their capacity – now and, as far as possible, over the next five years – and the vulnerability of their intended targets.

In each case, the question being asked is: how likely is it that this type of emergency will happen, somewhere in the country, sometime over the next five years. The NRA does not calculate the chances of these events happening in one particular place, or to one particular community or individual.

In terms of impact, the NRA takes account of the following effects:

- **The number of fatalities** that are directly attributable to the emergency.
- **Human illness or injury**, over a period following the onset of an emergency.
- **Social disruption** – the disruption to people's daily lives. Ten different types of disruption are taken into

account, from an inability to gain access to healthcare or schools, to interruptions in supplies of essential services like electricity or water, to the need for evacuation of individuals from an area.

- **Economic damage** – the effect on the economy overall, rather than the cost of repairs.

In addition, the NRA (but not – at present at least – Community Risk Registers) also attempts to estimate the psychological impact that emergencies may have. This includes the anxiety, loss of confidence or outrage that may be felt by communities throughout the country as a result of an emergency, or widespread changes to patterns of behaviour.[120]

2.2.3 Comparison of the risks

In planning for emergencies, local responders have to decide what types of risk, and what levels of consequence, to plan for. Putting a lot of effort into preparing for risks that are either very unlikely to happen, or are likely to cause relatively minor damage, is unlikely to be the best use of the time available to prepare. Priority is instead given to high risks: risks that are both relatively likely and could have a serious impact.

Apart from identifying the highest risks, the UK Government also provides guidance at national level and to

[120] United Kingdom's Cabinet Office (2008), 'National Risk Register', Available at: https://assets.publishing.service.gov.uk/government/uploads/system/uploads/attachment_data/file/61934/national_risk_register.pdf (accessed 24 August 2020).

Local Resilience Forums (LRFs) in England and Wales called planning assumptions, on the range and type of damage and disruption that might result from a selection of the higher risks. This ensures that planning is mostly non-specific and can be adapted to different scenarios when necessary.

At the national level the planning assumptions are used to set the parameters for the UK Resilience Capabilities Programme which co-ordinates planning and capability building for resilience across the UK.[121]

Although the three-step methodology the United Kingdom used to develop its national capability targets was able to successfully identify the potential accidents, natural events (hazards) and malicious attacks (threats) that could cause significant harm and disruption to the UK, there is little that is specific to the assessment of emerging public health threats at the national level.

2.3 Nigeria

The stages for assessing disaster risk in Nigeria are as follows:

Stage 1: Identifying specific disaster risk to be assessed.

Stage 2: Analysing disaster risk concerned.

Stage 3: Monitoring disaster risks.

---

[121] United Kingdom's Cabinet Office (2008), 'National Risk Register', Available at: https://assets.publishing.service.gov.uk/government/uploads/system/uploads/attachment_data/file/61934/national_risk_register.pdf (accessed 24 August 2020).

Stage 4: Evaluating disaster risk assessed, updating and disseminating information to all stakeholders.[122]

2.3.1 Identifying specific disaster risk(s)

This shall include:

i. Identifying the hazard.

ii. Describing the hazard (causes, frequency, magnitude, speed of onset, affected area and duration.[123]

2.3.2 Analysing the disaster risk(s)

This shall include:

i. Describing and quantifying vulnerability.

ii. Estimating likely losses resulting from the impact of hazard and disaster.

iii. Providing relevant hazard, vulnerability and risk maps.

iv. Identifying relevant capacities, methods and resources available to manage the risk.[124]

---

[122] Nigeria (2010), 'National disaster framework: Understanding the Framework', Available at: https://www.preventionweb.net/files/21708_nigherianationaldisastermanagementf.pdf (accessed 24 August 2020).

[123] Nigeria (2010), 'National disaster framework: Understanding the Framework', Available at: https://www.preventionweb.net/files/21708_nigherianationaldisastermanagementf.pdf (accessed 24 August 2020).

[124] Nigeria (2010), 'National disaster framework: Understanding the Framework', Available at: https://www.preventionweb.net/files/21708_nigherianationaldisastermanagementf.pdf (accessed 24 August 2020).

2.3.3 Monitoring Disaster Risks

All stakeholders shall have monitoring systems in place that are relevant to their specific functional responsibilities. This shall include monitoring of risks to ensure:

i. effectiveness of disaster risk reduction initiatives,

ii. changing patterns and new developments in risk profiles.[125]

2.3.4 Evaluating disaster risk assessed, updating and disseminating information to all stakeholders

This shall include:

i. Estimating the level of risk associated with a specific threat to determine whether the resulting risk is a priority or not.

ii. Prioritization of disaster risks when there are multiple threats to assess.

iii. Determining priority high risk people, households, areas, communities and infrastructures.

iv. Involving holistic and integrated planning and implementation in focussed disaster risk reduction initiatives.

[125] Nigeria (2010), 'National disaster framework: Understanding the Framework', Available at: https://www.preventionweb.net/files/21708_nigherianationaldisastermanagementf.pdf (accessed 24 August 2020).

v. Updating and disseminating risk assessment information.[126]

Although the four-step methodology Nigeria used to develop its national capability targets was able to successfully identify specific disaster risk to be assessed, there is little that is specific to the assessment of emerging public health threats at the national level.

The ensuing chapters provide further explanation of the risk assessment process for identifying, understanding, and reducing emerging and potential infectious threats to public health both nationally and internationally with the Financial Action Task Force risk assessment methodology.

[126] Nigeria (2010), 'National disaster framework: Understanding the Framework', Available at: https://www.preventionweb.net/files/21708_nigherianationaldisastermanagementf.pdf (accessed 24 August 2020).

CHAPTER 3

THE FINANCIAL ACTION TASK FORCE'S APPROACH TO NATIONAL RISK ASSESSMENT

Risk in the context of money laundering and terrorist financing is a function of three factors: ***threat, vulnerability*** **and** ***consequence***, and the money laundering and terrorist financing risks assessment involves making judgments about these 3 factors.[127]

A **threat** is anything, be it people, object or activity with the potential to cause harm to the country, society, or the economy. In the money laundering and terrorist financing context this includes criminals, their criminal activities, terrorist groups and their facilitators, their funds, as well as past, present and future money laundering or terrorist financing activities. Identifying the threat is an essential starting point in assessing money laundering and terrorist financing risks. It provides an

---

[127] Financial Action Task Force (2013), 'FATF Guidance: National money laundering and Terrorist Financing Risk Assessment', Available at: http://www.fatf-gafi.org/media/fatf/content/images/National_ML_TF_Risk_Assessment.pdf (accessed 27 July 2020).

understanding of the nature, size and volume of the predicate offences and proceeds of crimes and an understanding of the environment in which these offences are committed and the proceeds are generated.[128]

Vulnerability is what facilitates or creates the opportunity for money laundering. It may relate to a specific financial sector or product, or a weakness in regulation, supervision, or enforcement, or reflect unique circumstances in which it may be difficult to distinguish legal from illegal activity.[129]

Consequence refers to the impact or harm that money laundering or terrorist financing may cause and includes the effect of the underlying criminal and terrorist activity on financial systems and institutions.[130]

The risk-based approach is the standard approach for dealing with money laundering and terrorist financing.[131] The risk-based

---

[128] Yahaya, A. (2014), 'Encik Abu Hassan Alshari Yahaya: Results of the National Risk Assessment on money laundering and terrorist financing', Available at: https://www.bis.org/review/r141010c.pdf (accessed 6 June 2020).

[129] The US Treasury Department (2015), 'National Money Laundering Risk Assessment', Available at: https://www.treasury.gov/resource-center/terrorist-illicit-finance/Documents/National%20Money%20Laundering%20Risk%20Assessment%20%E2%80%93%2006-12-2015.pdf (accessed 6 June 2020).

[130] HM Treasury and Home Office (2015), 'UK national risk assessment of money laundering and terrorist financing', Available at: https://www.gov.uk/government/publications/uk-national-risk-assessment-of-money-laundering-and-terrorist-financing (accessed 6 June 2020).

[131] Financial Action Task Force (2012) (Updated 2019), 'INTERNATIONAL STANDARDS ON COMBATING MONEY LAUNDERING AND THE FINANCING OF TERRORISM & PROLIFERATION: The FATF Recommendations', Available at: http://www.fatf-gafi.org/media/fatf/documents/recommendations/pdfs/FATF%20Recommendations%202012.pdf (accessed 28 April 2020).

approach allows countries to adopt a more flexible set of measures, in order to target their resources more effectively and apply preventive measures that are commensurate to the nature of risks, in order to focus their efforts in the most effective way.[132]

Successful implementation of a risk-based approach to combating money-laundering and terrorist financing depends on a sound understanding of the threats and vulnerabilities. Where a country is seeking to introduce a risk-based approach at a national level, this will be greatly aided if there is a national understanding of the risks facing the country. This understanding can flow from a national risk assessment.[133]

3.1 NATIONAL RISK ASSESSMENT

The text of the Financial Action Task Force Recommendations (Recommendation 1) lays out a number of basic principles with regard to risk assessment. First, it calls on countries to "identify, assess and understand" the money laundering/terrorist financing (ML/TF) risks they face, and states that countries should also designate "an authority or mechanism to co-ordinate actions to assess risks". The goal of the standard is to ensure that countries can mitigate their ML/TF risks effectively, and the risk

---

[132] United States' Federal Financial Institutions Examination Council (2014), 'Bank Secrecy Act/Anti-Money Laundering Examination Manual', Available at: https://www.occ.treas.gov/publications/publications-by-type/other-publications-reports/ffiec-bsa-aml-examination-manual.pdf (accessed 10 January 2017).

[133] The Financial Action Task Force: Guidance on the Risk-Based Approach to Combating Money Laundering and Terrorist Financing 2007, para. 2.3.

assessment is clearly intended to serve as the basis for application of the risk-based approach, i.e., "to ensure that measures are commensurate with the risks identified." The text of the Recommendation adds that the "[risk-based] approach" (and therefore the risk assessment process on which it is based) should also be "an essential foundation" in allocating anti-money laundering and combating the financing of terrorism (AML/CFT) resources efficiently. Furthermore, the Recommendation indicates that risk assessments carried out by countries should be used for determining higher and lower risks that may then be addressed by applying enhanced measures or allowing simplified measures respectively.[134] The Recommendation concludes by requiring countries to assess risks "on an ongoing basis", and that they keep assessments up-to-date. The authority or mechanism designated to assess ML/TF risks in the country will likely be responsible for ensuring that this obligation is met. Recommendation 1, however, does not specify a particular period of time. Therefore, the frequency with which a risk assessment is updated is determined by the country, based on a number of factors,

[134] Financial Action Task Force (2012) (Updated 2019), 'INTERNATIONAL STANDARDS ON COMBATING MONEY LAUNDERING AND THE FINANCING OF TERRORISM & PROLIFERATION: The FATF Recommendations', Available at: http://www.fatf-gafi.org/media/fatf/documents/recommendations/pdfs/FATF%20Recommendations%202012.pdf (accessed 28 April 2020).

including how quickly (and how significantly) the risks may change.[135]

A national risk assessment should be regarded as a description of fundamental background information to assist supervisors, law enforcement authorities, the financial intelligence unit and financial institutions to ensure that decisions about allocating responsibilities and resources at the national level are based on a practical, comprehensive and up-to-date understanding of the risks.[136]

A national risk assessment should be tailored to the circumstances of the individual country, both in how it is executed, and its conclusions.[137] Countries should also consider how an understanding of the risks of money laundering and terrorist financing can be best achieved at the national level. Which body or bodies will be responsible for contributing to this assessment? How formal should an assessment be? Should the competent authority's view be made public? These are all questions for the competent authority to consider.[138]

---

135 Financial Action Task Force (2013), 'FATF Guidance: National money laundering and Terrorist Financing Risk Assessment', Available at: http://www.fatf-gafi.org/media/fatf/content/images/National_ML_TF_Risk_Assessment.pdf (accessed 27 July 2020).

136 The Financial Action Task Force: Guidance on the Risk-Based Approach to Combating Money Laundering and Terrorist Financing 2007, para. 2.23.

137 The Financial Action Task Force: Guidance on the Risk-Based Approach to Combating Money Laundering and Terrorist Financing 2007, para. 2.24.

138 The Financial Action Task Force: Guidance on the Risk-Based Approach to Combating Money Laundering and Terrorist Financing 2007, para. 2.25.

The desired outcome is that decisions about allocating responsibilities and resources at the national level are based on a comprehensive and up-to-date understanding of the risks. To achieve the desired outcome, competent authorities should develop and implement measures to mitigate the identified risks.[139]

The quality of the risk assessment exercise depends largely on the types and quality of data and information available. While quantitative assessments (*i.e.*, based mostly on statistics) may seem much more reliable and able to be replicated over time, the lack of available quantitative data in the ML/TF field makes it difficult to rely exclusively on such information. Moreover, information on all relevant factors may not be expressed or explained in numerical or quantitative form, and there is a danger that risk assessments relying heavily on available quantitative information may be biased towards risks that are easier to measure and discount those for which quantitative information is not readily available.[140]

For these reasons, it is advisable to complement an ML/TF risk assessment with relevant qualitative information such as, as appropriate, intelligence information, expert judgments, private sector input, case studies, thematic assessments, typologies

[139] The Financial Action Task Force: Guidance on the Risk-Based Approach to Combating Money Laundering and Terrorist Financing 2007, para. 2.26.
[140] Financial Action Task Force (2013), 'FATF Guidance: National money laundering and Terrorist Financing Risk Assessment', Available at: http://www.fatf-gafi.org/media/fatf/content/images/National_ML_TF_Risk_Assessment.pdf (accessed 27 July 2020).

studies and other (regional or supranational) risk assessments in addition to any available quantitative data. Similarly, objective data can be complemented by surveys or information of subjective nature such as perception indexes. Countries may in the long term wish to consider harmonising and further developing their quantitative data collection mechanisms that are used for ML/TF risk assessment in line with the FATF Standards (for example, Recommendation 33) and international best practices. It is essential that all participating organisations be authorised to share potentially sensitive information. Such information should be received, exchanged and used in accordance with agreed procedures, policies and applicable laws and regulations.[141]

Whatever form they take, a national assessment of the risks, along with measures to mitigate those risks, can inform how resources are applied to combat money laundering and terrorist financing, taking into account other relevant country policy goals. It can also inform how these resources are most effectively assigned to different public bodies, and how those bodies make use of their resources in an effective manner.[142]

As well as assisting competent authorities to decide how to allocate public funds to combat money laundering and terrorist

---

[141] Financial Action Task Force (2013), 'FATF Guidance: National money laundering and Terrorist Financing Risk Assessment', Available at: http://www.fatf-gafi.org/media/fatf/content/images/National_ML_TF_Risk_Assessment.pdf (accessed 27 July 2020).

[142] The Financial Action Task Force: Guidance on the Risk-Based Approach to Combating Money Laundering and Terrorist Financing 2007, para. 2.28.

financing, a national risk assessment can also inform decision makers about the relationship between the supervisory/regulatory regime and the identified risks. An over-zealous effort to counter the risks could be damaging and counter-productive, placing unreasonable burdens on industry, and act against the interests of the public by limiting access to financial services for some segments of the population. Alternatively, efforts may not be sufficient to provide protection to societies from the threats posed by criminals and terrorists. A sound understanding of the risks at the national level could help obviate these dangers.[143]

3.2 STAGES OF MONEY LAUNDERING NATIONAL RISK ASSESSMENT

The process of risk assessment can be divided into a series of activities or stages: *identification, analysis,* and *evaluation.* The three stages will be explained using the United Kingdom as a case study.

3.2.1 IDENTIFICATION

Risk identification is the process of finding, recognizing and describing risks. It is a screening exercise and serves as a preliminary step for the subsequent risk analysis stage. Risk analysis is the process to comprehend the nature of risk and to determine the level of risk. Risk evaluation is the process of

[143] The Financial Action Task Force: Guidance on the Risk-Based Approach to Combating Money Laundering and Terrorist Financing 2007, para. 2.29.

comparing the results of risk analysis with risk criteria to determine whether the risk and/or its magnitude is acceptable or tolerable.[144]

In general terms, the process of *identification* in the context of an ML/TF risk assessment starts by developing an initial list of potential risks or risk factors countries face when combating ML/TF. These will be drawn from known or suspected threats or vulnerabilities. Ideally at this stage, the identification process should attempt to be comprehensive; however, it should also be dynamic in the sense that new or previously undetected risks identified may also be considered at any stage in the process.[145]

Risk identification should be based as much as possible on quantitative (historical, statistical) data. However, as the purpose of the risk identification stage is to find and recognize all likely hazards and significant consequences, it is appropriate to extensively use also qualitative methods, such as expert opinions, intelligence information, check-lists, systematic team approaches, inductive reasoning techniques, or other. Techniques to improve the completeness of the risk identification process may also include brainstorming and

---

144 European Commission (2010), 'Risk Assessment and Mapping Guidelines for Disaster Management', Available at: https://ec.europa.eu/echo/files/about/COMM_PDF_SEC_2010_1626_F_staff_working_document_en.pdf (accessed 29 July 2020).

145 Financial Action Task Force (2013), 'FATF Guidance: National money laundering and Terrorist Financing Risk Assessment', Available at: http://www.fatf-gafi.org/media/fatf/content/images/National_ML_TF_Risk_Assessment.pdf (accessed 27 July 2020).

Delphi methodology (interactive forecasting method relying on a panel of experts).[146]

The first stage of the United Kingdom's national risk assessment of money laundering and terrorist financing, identification, focused on gathering information through consultation with a broad range of stakeholders. This was in order to identify vulnerabilities and threats. Firstly the United Kingdom (UK) held a series of workshops and bilateral meetings with a broad range of stakeholders including firms and industry representatives from the sectors subject to the Money Laundering Regulations, law enforcement agencies, supervisory authorities, other government departments and non-governmental organisations (NGOs).

Previous assessments conducted by law enforcement and other bodies were used to assist in identifying the main threats to the UK. Business activities presenting risk were identified and prioritised according to the level of risk. Workshops were held with some sectors and questionnaires issued to others. In addition to the annual reporting process for supervisors, they were each asked to complete a questionnaire specifically for this assessment.[147]

---

[146] European Commission (2010), 'Risk Assessment and Mapping Guidelines for Disaster Management', Available at: https://ec.europa.eu/echo/files/about/COMM_PDF_SEC_2010_1626_F_staff_working_document_en.pdf (accessed 29 July 2020).

[147] HM Treasury and Home Office (2015), 'UK national risk assessment of money laundering and terrorist financing', Available at:

3.2.2 ANALYSIS

Risk analysis is the process to comprehend the nature of risk and to determine the level of risk. For every risk and risk scenario identified in the previous risk identification stage, the risk analysis process carries out a detailed (and if possible quantitative) estimation of the probability of its occurrence and the severity of the potential impacts.[148]

Analysis lies at the heart of the ML/TF risk assessment process. It involves consideration of the nature, sources, likelihood and consequences of the identified risks or risk factors. Ultimately, the aim of this stage is to gain a holistic understanding of each of the risks – as a combination of threat, vulnerability and consequence in order to work toward assigning some sort of relative value or importance to them. Risk analysis can be undertaken with varying degrees of detail, depending on the type of risk and the purpose of the risk assessment, as well as based on the information, data and resources available.[149]

https://www.gov.uk/government/publications/uk-national-risk-assessment-of-money-laundering-and-terrorist-financing (accessed 24 August 2020).

148 European Commission (2010), 'Risk Assessment and Mapping Guidelines for Disaster Management', Available at: https://ec.europa.eu/echo/files/about/COMM_PDF_SEC_2010_1626_F_staff_working_document_en.pdf (accessed 29 July 2020).

149 Financial Action Task Force (2013), 'FATF Guidance: National money laundering and Terrorist Financing Risk Assessment', Available at: http://www.fatf-gafi.org/media/fatf/content/images/National_ML_TF_Risk_Assessment.pdf (accessed 27 July 2020).

It is important during risk analysis to establish the geographic scope of the risk scenario and of the impacts, even though the precise location may be left unspecified. In more advanced national risk assessments, a greater number of risks in localized areas on the national territory, such as a river basin or a city, depending on the hazard and the level of analysis, should be considered, if possible. Keeping track of the local dimension of risks is important to avoid possible double-counting of impacts; and may help avoiding possible omissions.[150]

The second stage of the UK's national risk assessment of money laundering and terrorist financing involved analysing the data provided by stakeholders to establish the risks present, and understand their impact. Given the largely hidden nature of money laundering and terrorist financing, the data used for this assessment was regarded in certain places as being partial, inconsistent or contradictory. The conclusions of the UK's national risk assessment of money laundering and terrorist financing draws heavily on expert judgment from law enforcement agencies, supervisory authorities and those responsible for anti-money laundering and combating the financing of terrorism (AML/CFT) within firms.

[150] European Commission (2010), 'Risk Assessment and Mapping Guidelines for Disaster Management', Available at: https://ec.europa.eu/echo/files/about/COMM_PDF_SEC_2010_1626_F_staff_working_document_en.pdf (accessed 29 July 2020).

The risks identified were tested through a peer review process with stakeholders. Peer review workshops were conducted on a sector by sector basis, including industry representatives, supervisors and law enforcement agencies. Stakeholders were invited to submit any necessary additional information to support their views.

As a result, the UK's national risk assessment of money laundering and terrorist financing represents the broad views of all those participating in the UK's AML/CFT regime from regulated firms in the private sector, to police forces and national law enforcement agencies, government departments and supervisory authorities. It also reflects input from leading NGOs in this area including Global Witness and Transparency International.[151]

3.2.3 EVALUATION

Risk evaluation is the process of comparing the results of risk analysis with risk criteria to determine whether the risk and/or its magnitude is acceptable or tolerable. Risk criteria are the terms of reference against which the significance of a risk is evaluated. The risk criteria may include associated costs and benefits, legal requirements, socioeconomic and environmental factors, concerns of stakeholders, etc. Risk evaluation is used to

151 HM Treasury and Home Office (2015), 'UK national risk assessment of money laundering and terrorist financing', Available at: https://www.gov.uk/government/publications/uk-national-risk-assessment-of-money-laundering-and-terrorist-financing (accessed 24 August 2020).

make decisions about the significance of risks whether each specific risk should be accepted or treated. The International Risk Governance Council (2006) describes the objectives of risk evaluation as a judgement on the reliability and acceptability based on balancing pros and cons, testing potential impacts on quality of life, discussing different development options for the economy and society and weighing the competing arguments and evidence claims in a balanced way.[152]

Evaluation in the context of the ML/TF risk assessment process involves taking the risks analysed during the previous stage to determine priorities for addressing them, taking into account the purpose established at the beginning of the assessment process. These priorities can contribute to development of a strategy for their mitigation.[153]

The final stage of the UK's national risk assessment of money laundering and terrorist financing was the evaluation of the relative exposure of each sector to risk. As part of this, areas were ranked on the basis of risk, using a model developed from the National Crime Agency's draft Management of Risk in Law Enforcement (MoRiLE), which

---

[152] European Commission (2010), 'Risk Assessment and Mapping Guidelines for Disaster Management', Available at: https://ec.europa.eu/echo/files/about/COMM_PDF_SEC_2010_1626_F_staff_working_document_en.pdf (accessed 29 July 2020).

[153] Financial Action Task Force (2013), 'FATF Guidance: National money laundering and Terrorist Financing Risk Assessment', Available at: http://www.fatf-gafi.org/media/fatf/content/images/National_ML_TF_Risk_Assessment.pdf (accessed 27 July 2020).

was amended to reduce the dependency on quantitative data and include factors for qualitative assessment. The methodologies used by the World Bank and International Monetary Fund were also considered during the development phase. The terrorist financing risks were assessed separately.[154]

The UK's national risk assessment risk rating model assesses the structural risk within each area, based on a series of factors to indicate the vulnerability of a particular sector to money laundering and the relative likelihood that the threat of money laundering will materialise in that particular sector, given there is general threat to the UK that criminals will attempt to launder money through some means.

It should also be noted that this model focuses on the risk of businesses in a sector being used by criminals to facilitate money laundering, wittingly or unwittingly, due to the services it offers, rather than the risk that business itself is established as a front for money laundering. The risks with regard to criminal spend, or the use of the business itself to conceal money laundering, may be substantially different.[155]

---

[154] HM Treasury and Home Office (2015), 'UK national risk assessment of money laundering and terrorist financing', Available at: https://www.gov.uk/government/publications/uk-national-risk-assessment-of-money-laundering-and-terrorist-financing (accessed 24 August 2020).

[155] HM Treasury and Home Office (2015), 'UK national risk assessment of money laundering and terrorist financing', Available at: https://www.gov.uk/government/publications/uk-national-risk-assessment-of-money-laundering-and-terrorist-financing (accessed 24 August 2020).

The assessment had also looked at means of transferring funds that provide a degree of anonymity, and so present a greater risk than payments through the conventional payment systems that are directly linked to a bank account, such as debit/credit card payments, direct debit or other transactions through bank payment systems.

A range of factors were considered when assessing the risk within the sectors, including law enforcement agencies' existing knowledge of money laundering through the sector, where a lower level of knowledge represents a vulnerability and so a higher level of risk.

The factors considered when assessing the vulnerability of a particular sector or area include:

- the relative complexity and reach (national/ international) of the services offered by the sector, or the capacity to move money internationally given the nature of the funds (i.e. cash, e-money);
- the relative volume and speed of money movement through firms in the sector, or the volume and speed of money movement given the nature of the funds;
- the level of compliance within the sector a higher level of risk.

For factors such as complexity, reach and volume, and speed of money movement the ratings are based on the nature of business undertaken by the majority of the sector.

The factors considered when assessing the likelihood that a threat will materialise in a particular sector/area include:

- the size of the sector or area;
- the likelihood that the sector will report suspicious activity to law enforcement, as indicated by the level of suspicious activity report (SAR) submission by the sector;
- law enforcement agencies' existing knowledge of money laundering through the sector.

The consequences of criminals successfully laundering money through a particular sector were assumed to be severe for all the areas covered.

Following the scoring of vulnerabilities and likelihoods, the matrix produces a score for the thematic area's risk, which is then categorised into Low, Medium or High risk levels. The model then considers the mitigating measures in place in terms of UK law enforcement agencies and supervisors' capability and capacity to combat money laundering in that area. The combined mitigation score has the potential to reduce the overall risk level of a thematic area where law enforcement/supervisory activity effectively mitigates the risk. Once applied, an overall risk score for the thematic area is calculated and then categorised.[156]

---

156 HM Treasury and Home Office (2015), 'UK national risk assessment of money laundering and terrorist financing', Available at: https://www.gov.uk/government/publications/uk-national-risk-assessment-of-money-laundering-and-terrorist-financing (accessed 24 August 2020).

CHAPTER 4

ASSESSING THE RISKS OF EMERGING INFECTIOUS DISEASES WITH THE FINANCIAL ACTION TASK FORCE RISK ASSESSMENT STRATEGY

The previous chapter explained the risk assessment process for identifying and managing money laundering/terrorist financing risks (identification, analysis, and evaluation). This chapter will explain how countries can identify, analyse, and evaluate emerging and potential infectious threats to public health both nationally and internationally using the Financial Action Task Force risk assessment strategy with a focus on COVID-19.

4.1. First stage: identification

A first step of the risk assessment exercise is for a country to identify both local and international risks. A good foundation for the identification process is to begin by compiling a list of the major known or suspected threats and vulnerabilities that exist both locally and internationally. The identified threats or vulnerabilities should of course relate to the purpose and scope of the assessment and this will also influence whether they are more micro or macro in focus.[157]

Formulating a list of a country's emerging and potential infectious threats to public health both nationally and internationally will require the collective knowledge of the relevant authorities involved in combating infectious diseases in the country. Situation and project reports from hospitals and the country's Centre for Disease Control, and reports from both the Federal and State Ministry of Health will help in the compilation of this list. Thus, discussion of the threat of infectious diseases will probably need involvement of appropriate experts who contribute to compiling this initial list of the main or common threats and vulnerabilities of newly discovered diseases.

For infectious diseases threats from foreign jurisdictions, the development of a list may be facilitated by having access to information from the World Health Organization and the United States Centers for Disease Control and Prevention. Most countries around the world have designated Centers for Disease Control and Prevention (CDC). The CDC works 24/7 to protect its citizens from health, safety and security threats, both foreign and locally. Whether diseases start at home or abroad,

157 Financial Action Task Force (2013), 'FATF GUIDANCE: National Money Laundering and Terrorist Financing Risk Assessment', Available at: https://www.fatf-gafi.org/documents/documents/nationalmoneylaunderingandterroristfinancingriskassessment.html (accessed 27 April 2020).

are chronic or acute, curable or preventable, human error or deliberate attack, CDC fights diseases and supports communities and citizens to do the same. Most importantly, CDC conducts critical science and provides health information that protects the nation against expensive and dangerous health threats, and responds when these arise.[158]

International risks can also be identified using standard due diligence measures like desk-based research. Desk-based research will help countries to identify jurisdictions with infectious diseases. Desk-based research may require competent authorities in various countries to continuously monitor the news regularly for any new developments regarding strange diseases. Countries may monitor the news by watching television stations like the Cable News Network (CNN), Sky News and British Broadcasting Corporation (BBC) or alternatively carrying out extensive research on the internet for news about current outbreaks or incidents of potential new and emerging infectious diseases in animals or humans, occurring anywhere in the world. If a country through the desk-based research discovers the presence of a disease in another country, the Country must then take note of the name of the disease and the exact location of the disease; the disease may be present in more than one country.

[158] United States Centers for Disease Control and Prevention (2020), 'Mission, Role and Pledge', Available at: https://www.cdc.gov/about/organization/mission.htm (accessed 27 April 2020).

As it relates to COVID-19, available evidence suggests that the cluster was initially reported on 31 December 2019, when the World Health Organization (WHO) China Country Office was informed of cases of pneumonia of unknown etiology (unknown cause) detected in Wuhan City, Hubei Province of China, and this information was made available in the WHO website for countries to see. As of 3 January 2020, a total of 44 patients with pneumonia of unknown etiology had been reported to WHO by the national authorities in China. Of the 44 cases reported, 11 were severely ill, while the remaining 33 patients were in stable condition. According to media reports, the concerned market in Wuhan was closed on 1 January 2020 for environmental sanitation and disinfection. The causal agent had not yet been identified or confirmed. On 1 January 2020, WHO requested further information from national authorities to assess the risk.[159]

On 11 and 12 January 2020, WHO received further detailed information from the Chinese National Health Commission about the outbreak. The evidence was highly suggestive that the outbreak is associated with exposures in one seafood market in Wuhan. The market was closed on 1 January 2020. At this stage, there was no infection among

159 World Health Organization (2020), 'Pneumonia of unknown cause – China', Available at: https://www.who.int/csr/don/05-january-2020-pneumonia-of-unkown-cause-china/en/ (accessed 27 April 2020).

healthcare workers, and no clear evidence of human to human transmission.[160]

Countries who received the above information from the WHO should have immediately taking note of the name of the disease (COVID-19) and the exact location which is China.

4.2. Second stage: analysis

Having identified local and international risk(s) at the standard due diligence stage, Countries should conduct further studies on the severity and transmissibility of the virus to determine if the virus can be transmitted from one person to another person or if it can only be from Animals to Human Beings.[161] This research will advance scientific understanding of the virus and contribute to the development of medical countermeasures such as vaccines and treatments.

Countries can send a team of medical experts to the country affected, to elicit more information about the identified risks. This may be done personally or through an international agency like the World Health Organization.

---

[160] World Health Organization (2020), 'Novel Coronavirus – China', Available at: https://www.who.int/csr/don/12-january-2020-novel-coronavirus-china/en/ (accessed 28 April 2020).

[161] Financial Action Task Force (2013), 'FATF Guidance: National Money Laundering and Terrorist Financing Risk Assessment', Available at: https://www.fatf-gafi.org/documents/documents/nationalmoneylaunderingandterroristfinancingriskassessment.html (accessed 27 April 2020).

On 20-21 January 2020, a World Health Organization (WHO) delegation conducted a field visit to Wuhan to learn about the response to 2019 novel coronavirus (2019-nCOV). The mission was part of the on-going close collaboration between WHO and Chinese national, provincial, and Wuhan health authorities in responding to 2019-nCoV.

The delegation visited the Wuhan Tianhe Airport, Zhongnan hospital, Hubei provincial CDC, including the BSL3 laboratory in China's Center for Disease Control (CDC). The delegation observed and discussed active surveillance processes, temperature screening at the airport, laboratory facilities, infection prevention and control measures at the hospital and its associated fever clinics, and the deployment of the rRT-PCR test kit to detect the virus.

Data collected through detailed epidemiological investigation and through the deployment of the new test kit nationally revealed that human-to-human transmission is taking place in Wuhan.[162]

On 22 January 2020, the meeting of the Emergency Committee convened by the WHO Director-General under the International Health Regulations (IHR) (2005) regarding the outbreak of novel coronavirus 2019 in the People's Republic of China, with exportations currently reported in the Republic of Korea, Japan, Thailand and Singapore, took place. Chinese authorities presented

---

162 World Health Organization (2020), 'Mission summary: WHO Field Visit to Wuhan, China 20-21 January 2020', Available at: https://www.who.int/china/news/detail/22-01-2020-field-visit-wuhan-china-jan-2020 (accessed 28 April 2020).

new epidemiological information that revealed an increase in the number of cases, of suspected cases, of affected provinces, and the proportion of deaths in currently reported cases of 4% (17 of 557). They reported fourth-generation cases in Wuhan and second-generation cases outside Wuhan, as well as some clusters outside Hubei province.[163]

On 30 January 2020, the second meeting of the Emergency Committee convened by the WHO Director-General under the International Health Regulations (IHR) (2005) regarding the outbreak of novel coronavirus 2019 in the People's Republic of China, with exportations to other countries, took place. Representatives of the Ministry of Health of the People's Republic of China reported on the current situation and the public health measures being taken. According to the Representatives there are now 7711 confirmed and 12167 suspected cases throughout the country. Of the confirmed cases, 1370 are severe and 170 people had died. 124 people had recovered and been discharged from hospital.[164]

---

[163] World Health Organization (2020), 'Statement on the meeting of the International Health Regulations (2005) Emergency Committee regarding the outbreak of novel coronavirus (2019-nCoV)', Available at: https://www.who.int/news-room/detail/23-01-2020-statement-on-the-meeting-of-the-international-health-regulations-(2005)-emergency-committee-regarding-the-outbreak-of-novel-coronavirus-(2019-ncov) (accessed 28 April 2020).

[164] World Health Organization (2020), 'Statement on the second meeting of the International Health Regulations (2005) Emergency Committee regarding the outbreak of novel coronavirus (2019-nCoV)', Available at: https://www.who.int/news-room/detail/30-01-2020-statement-on-the-second-meeting-of-the-international-health-regulations-(2005)-emergency-committee-regarding-the-outbreak-of-novel-coronavirus-(2019-ncov) (accessed 28 April 2020).

4.3. Third stage: evaluation

The last stage of risk assessment is evaluation. It involves taking the results found during the analysis process to determine priorities for addressing the risks.[165] Where countries identify higher risks, they should ensure that their regime addresses these higher risks by applying a risk-based approach to ensure that measures to prevent or mitigate risks are commensurate with the risks identified but where countries identify lower risks, they should apply simplified measures.[166] For example, if the risk analysis had revealed that the disease or diseases cannot be transmitted from one person to another person but only from Animals to Human Beings then countries will classify the risk as low risk or medium risk but where it is determined that the disease or diseases can be easily transmitted from person to person then countries must classify the risk as high risk.

Proportionate procedures should be designed based on assessed risk(s). Infectious diseases should be subject to enhanced procedures while non-infectious diseases should be subject to

165 Financial Action Task Force (2013), 'FATF Guidance: National Money Laundering and Terrorist Financing Risk Assessment', Available at: https://www.fatf-gafi.org/documents/documents/nationalmoneylaunderingandterroristfinancingriskassessment.html (accessed 27 April 2020).

166 Financial Action Task Force (2012), 'International Standards on Combating Money Laundering and the Financing of Terrorism and Proliferation (The FATF Recommendations)', Available at: https://www.fatf-gafi.org/publications/fatfrecommendations/documents/internationalstandardsoncombatingmoneylaunderingandthefinancingofterrorismproliferation-thefatfrecommendations.html (accessed 6 May 2020).

standard procedures.[167] Proportionate procedures will vary according to the extent of a country's leverage in addressing the risk(s). Countries can use the **National capacities review tool**, recommended by the World Health Organization, to determine if it has leverage to prevent or mitigate risk. The National capacities review tool will determine the following:

i. *Which coronaviruses (CoV) diagnostic tests is the country capable of conducting?*
ii. *Does the country have the ability to quickly enhance current surveillance?*
iii. *Is there a functioning respiratory disease surveillance system in place or pneumonia surveillance systems?*
iv. *Is the private sector included in the respiratory surveillance system?*
v. *Do the public health staff at local/regional and/or national levels have the skills to analyze the surveillance data to detect SARI/pneumonia outbreaks/clusters?*
vi. *Are there Public Health Rapid Response Teams (RRTs) available in the country?*
vii. *How are RRTs identified and assigned when alerts are identified?*
viii. *Are RRT trained specifically in contact tracing?*

---

[167] Financial Action Task Force (2007), 'FATF Guidance on the Risk-Based Approach to Combating Money Laundering and Terrorist Financing - High Level Principles and Procedures', Available at: https://www.fatf-gafi.org/publications/fatfrecommendations/documents/fatfguidanceontherisk-basedapproachtocombatingmoneylaunderingandterroristfinancing-highlevelprinciplesandprocedures.html (accessed 6 May, 2020).

ix. *Are RRT trained in biological sample collection for respiratory pathogens?*

x. *Does the country have surge capacity for contact tracing?*

xi. *Does the country have tools to follow up cases and contacts?*

xii. *Does the country have a national public health emergency preparedness and response plan that can address respiratory diseases including novel coronaviruses?*

xiii. *Does an Emergency operation Center (EOC)/Incident Management Structure (IMS) exist in the country?*

xiv. *Is there a team of risk communication, communications or health promotion professionals at the national and subnational levels who are trained in risk communication and can be called upon to design and implement risk communication strategies during crises? Is there surge support available within the government, in partner agencies or elsewhere to cover increased communication needs during a public health crisis*

xv. *Are staff working at Point of Entry (PoE) aware of the appropriate action to manage ill passenger(s) detected before boarding, on board conveyances (such as planes and ships) and on arrival at PoE?*

xvi. *Is there an appropriate place for rapid health assessment and isolation, in the event of detecting a potential nCoV case at PoE?*

xvii. *Is there a mechanism for safely transporting ill travelers to designated hospitals, including the identification of adequate ambulance services?*

xviii. *Is there a functioning Infection Prevention and Control (IPC) program in each hospital/health care facility in the area where cases are suspected/identified/transferred?*[168]

Answers to the above questions will help a country in formulating a list of its major vulnerabilities to infectious diseases. The list will help a country to determine if it can afford to manage the newly found disease or if it should avoid the disease completely due to lack of adequate resources and manpower.

If majority of the questions above are answered in the negative then countries will have to avoid the risk completely, and in the context of COVID-19 this will mean officially shutting the country's airports, seaports, and borders while stillimplementing a full lockdown—involving the closure of schools and non-essential workplaces and a ban on social gatherings. But if majority of the questions are answered in the affirmative Countries should implement necessary measures and allocate appropriate resources to mitigate the risks which they have identified, and this includes aggressive testing and contact

[168] World Health Organization (2020), 'National capacities review tool for a novel coronavirus (nCoV)', Available at: https://www.who.int/publications/i/item/national-capacities-review-tool-for-a-novelcoronavirus (accessed 27 April 2020).

tracing, combined with medical countermeasures such as vaccines and treatments.[169]

The experience of China, the Republic of Korea, Singapore and others clearly demonstrates that aggressive testing and contact tracing, combined with social distancing measures and community mobilization, can prevent infections and save lives.[170] If countries detect, test, treat, isolate, trace, and mobilize their people in the response, those with a handful of cases can prevent those cases becoming clusters, and those clusters becoming community transmission.[171]

Where a country lacks the capacity to manage the threat of infectious diseases but still decides to accept the risk(s), the consequences may be severe. For example, at midday on March 17, a week after the World Health Organisation declared the novel coronavirus a pandemic and 20 days after Nigeria reported its index case, Dr. Chikwe Ihekweazu, the Director General of the Nigeria Centre for Disease Control

169 Financial Action Task Force (2013), 'FATF Guidance: National Money Laundering and Terrorist Financing Risk Assessment', Available at: https://www.fatf-gafi.org/documents/documents/nationalmoneylaunderingandterroristfinancingriskassessment.html (accessed 27 April 2020).

170 World Health Organization (2020), 'WHO Director-General's opening remarks at the media briefing on COVID-19', Available at: https://www.who.int/dg/speeches/detail/who-director-general-s-opening-remarks-at-the-mission-briefing-on-covid-19---13-march-2020 (accessed 27 April 2020).

171 World Health Organization (2020), 'WHO Director-General's opening remarks at the media briefing on COVID-19', Available at: https://www.who.int/dg/speeches/detail/who-director-general-s-opening-remarks-at-the-media-briefing-on-covid-19---11-march-2020 (accessed 27 April 2020).

(NCDC) called a meeting of top medical experts to appraise the country's preparedness. During the appraisal of Nigeria's readiness, the meeting revealed that Nigeria had an estimated 350 intensive care units for 200 million people, according to officials present. Experts estimated Nigeria's hospitals with Intensive Care Units (ICU) infrastructure at 71, with each having between one to 20 beds. The total number of ICU beds in the country was put at 350.[172]

A report from the Punch Newspapers revealed that as at March 24, 2020, Nigeria did not have up to 500 ventilators across the 36 states and the Federal Capital Territory.[173] This information was corroborated by the President of the Nigerian Medical Association who confirmed that Nigeria does not have enough ventilators.[174]

The Nigeria Centre for Disease Control had also shown through the way it handled the first index case of COVID-

---

[172] Premium Times (2020), 'Coronavirus: Nigeria has 350 ICU beds for 200 million people', Available at: https://www.premiumtimesng.com/news/headlines/384840-coronavirus-nigeria-has-350-icu-beds-for-200-million-people.html (accessed 30 April 2020).

[173] The Punch (2020), 'Nigeria has less than 500 ventilators for coronavirus patients — Sources', Available at: https://punchng.com/nigeria-has-less-than-500-ventilators-for-coronavirus-patients-sources/ (accessed 28 April 2020).

[174] Anglican Cable Network Nigeria (2020), 'FG, Minister Ignored Advice On Coronavirus Containment — NMA', Available at: https://acnntv.com/fg-minister-ignored-advice-on-coronavirus-containment-nma/ (accessed 28 April 2020).

19 that it had difficulty with tracing the contacts of the index case.[175]

Despite the numerous challenges faced by the Nigerian health sector as highlighted above, the Federal Government as of March 17, 2020 said that it had no plans to impose travel restrictions on visitors from countries where coronavirus continued to spread rapidly.[176] The Federal Government had decided to screen visitors entering the country from China (where the disease originated last year), Japan, Iran, Italy, Germany, France, South Korea and Spain.[177] It was not until the 21st of March 2020 that the government through the Presidential Task Force on the Coronavirus placed travel restrictions on entry into the country from 13 countries with high-burden of coronavirus. The countries are China, Iran, South Korea, Germany, Italy, United States, United Kingdom, Switzerland, Norway, Netherlands, Spain, France, and Japan.[178] This measure proved ineffective as Nigeria had recorded 14 new cases of

---

[175] Nigeria Centre for Disease Control (2020), 'COVID-19 OUTBREAK IN NIGERIA: Situation Report', Available at: https://www.ncdc.gov.ng/themes/common/files/sitreps/3f45aa7d759bfc31a928a56470?8720c.pdf (accessed 28 April 2020).

[176] The Punch (2020), 'No stopping Chinese, Italians, others from visiting Nigeria — FG', Available at: https://punchng.com/no-stopping-chinese-italians-others-from-visiting-nigeria-fg/ (accessed 28 April 2020).

[177] The Punch (2020), 'No stopping Chinese, Italians, others from visiting Nigeria — FG', Available at: https://punchng.com/no-stopping-chinese-italians-others-from-visiting-nigeria-fg/ (accessed 28 April 2020).

[178] The Punch (2020), 'UPDATED: FG places travel ban on China, Italy, US, UK, nine others', Available at: https://punchng.com/breaking-fg-places-travel-ban-on-china-italy-us-uk-others/ (accessed 28 April 2020).

coronavirus, bringing the total number of infections to 111 in the country as of March 29, 2020; the reason could be that people from high-risk countries were still able to enter Nigeria through low risk jurisdictions.[179]

As of 7 March 2020, the global number of confirmed cases of COVID-19 had surpassed 100,000.[180] On the 11th of March 2020, the World Health Organization made the assessment that COVID-19 can be characterized as a pandemic in view of the fact that the number of cases of COVID-19 outside China had increased 13-fold, and the number of affected countries had tripled. There were now more than 118,000 cases in 114 countries, and 4,291 people had lost their lives. Thousands more were fighting for their lives in hospitals.[181] As of 13 March 2020, more than 132,000 cases of COVID-19 had now been reported to WHO, from 123 countries and territories. Europe had now become the epicenter of the pandemic, with more reported cases and deaths than the rest of the world combined, apart

[179] The Punch (2020), 'UPDATED: Nigeria reports 14 new coronavirus cases, total now 111', Available at: https://punchng.com/breaking-nigeria-reports-14-new-cases-total-at-111/ (accessed 30 April 2020).

[180] World Health Organization (2020), 'WHO statement on cases of COVID-19 surpassing 100 000', Available at: https://www.who.int/news-room/detail/07-03-2020-who-statement-on-cases-of-covid-19-surpassing-100-000 (accessed 28 April 2020).

[181] World Health Organization (2020), 'WHO Director-General's opening remarks at the media briefing on COVID-19', Available at: https://www.who.int/dg/speeches/detail/who-director-general-s-opening-remarks-at-the-media-briefing-on-covid-19---11-march-2020 (accessed 27 April 2020).

from China.[182] Despite this information, the Federal Government waited till the 29th of March 2020 to shut the country's airports, seaports, and borders. As of March 29 when the President of Nigeria shut the country's airports, seaports, and borders, Nigeria had recorded 111 confirmed cases of COVID-19 and one death.[183]

The best approach would have been for the Federal Government to have avoided the COVID-19 risk in its entirety since it lacked the leverage to accept and mitigate the risks. This will be done through the closure of the country's borders, seaport, and airports. Nigerian citizens who desired to come into Nigeria from other jurisdictions should still be allowed to come in on the condition that they are tested for COVID-19 and certified negative before boarding the plane. Even after testing negative, they should be placed under mandatory quarantine for 15 days upon arrival. This will allow medical personnel to carry out further tests to verify if they are indeed COVID-19 negative. The mandatory quarantine should be done in a place very close to the airport; It can be a hotel. These measures would have been able to limit the spread of the virus in Nigeria, and averted a total lockdown of the country.

---

182 World Health Organization (2020), 'WHO Director-General's opening remarks at the media briefing on COVID-19', Available at: https://www.who.int/dg/speeches/detail/who-director-general-s-opening-remarks-at-the-mission-briefing-on-covid-19---13-march-2020 (accessed 28 March 2020).

183 The Punch (2020), 'Sanwo-Olu blames late airport, border closure for COVID-19 spread', Available at: https://punchng.com/sanwo-olu-blames-late-airport-border-closure-for-covid-19-spread/ (accessed 30 April 2020).

CHAPTER 5

RISK CONTROL MEASURES

The goal of risk control measures is to interrupt direct human-to-human transmission. Where countries discover through the Financial Action Task Force National Risk Assessment Process that human-to-human transmission is taking place in the jurisdiction concerned, they should ensure that their regime adequately addresses such risks. But where data collected through detailed epidemiological investigation and through the deployment of new test kits nationally suggests that no human-to-human transmission is taking place in the jurisdiction concerned, countries may decide to allow simplified measures under certain conditions. This approach should be an essential foundation to efficient allocation of resources across the public health sector and the implementation of risk-based medical countermeasures.

Outbreak control activities are based on the early identification and systematic rapid isolation of cases under appropriate Infection Prevention and Control (IPC) measures, timely and comprehensive contact tracing, disinfection of infectious materials and the appropriate use of personal protective equipment. Isolation of infected patients with appropriate IPC measures has been shown to effectively stop the spread of disease in previous outbreaks.

Appropriate resources are needed to monitor risk assessment strategies in terms of their efficacy. This means that the assessments should be able to identify the risks and issues, properly assess their level of importance, and ensure that appropriate remedies are in place.

This chapter will expound on the measures that can help curb the spread of infectious diseases with a primary focus on COVID-19.

5.1 REDUCING THE SPREAD OF DISEASE: INFECTION CONTROL & RESPIRATORY AND HAND HYGIENE

COVID-19 can spread from person to person via the respiratory route when an infected person coughs and sneezes, and through hand-to-face (nose, mouth or eye) contact after a person or surface that is contaminated with infectious respiratory droplets has been touched. Visitors and residents in affected areas are at low risk of becoming infected in the community if the precautionary measures below are followed:

- Stay at home.
- avoid contact with symptomatic patients/their bodily fluids, corpses and/or bodily fluids from deceased patients

- avoid consumption of bush meat and contact with wild animals, both alive and dead
- wash and peel fruit and vegetables before consumption
- Adopt thorough respiratory and hand hygiene practices, i.e. covering the nose and mouth with a tissue when coughing and sneezing, disposing immediately of that tissue after use, and washing hands frequently with soap and warm water, or alcohol gel if water is not readily available.; and
- ensure safe sexual practices.[184]

It is advisable to avoid habitats that may be populated by bats, such as caves or mines in areas/countries where COVID-19 has been reported, as well as any form of close contact with wild animals, including monkeys, forest antelopes, rodents and bats, both alive and dead, and manipulation or consumption of any type of bushmeat.[185]

---

[184] European Centre for Disease Prevention and Control. Rapid risk assessment: Ebola virus disease outbreak in North Kivu and Ituri Provinces, Democratic Republic of the Congo – fourth update – 16 April 2019. ECDC: Stockholm; 2019.

[185] European Centre for Disease Prevention and Control. Factsheet about Ebola and Marburg fevers [Internet]. Stockholm: ECDC; 2016 [cited 11 April 2019]. Available from: http://ecdc.europa.eu/ebola-and-marburg-fevers/facts/factsheet (accessed 31 July 2020).

5.2 INTERNATIONAL TRAVEL, BORDER RESTRICTIONS AND SCREENING

To reduce the likelihood of infectious diseases being introduced into a particular country, the following options for response can be considered:

- Where exit screening is implemented at an airport, a traveller presenting with symptoms (e.g. fever >38°C) should not be allowed to board a flight.[186]
- A passenger who develops COVID-19-compatible symptoms while on board a commercial flight should be isolated and his/her condition ascertained upon arrival. Should the passenger be confirmed as having COVID-19, contact tracing of passengers should be initiated in accordance with the recommendations for aircraft contact tracing set out in the European Centre for Disease Prevention and Control (ECDC) Risk assessment guidelines for infectious diseases transmitted on aircraft (RAGIDA).[187]

186 European Centre for Disease Prevention and Control. (2019), 'Rapid risk assessment: Ebola virus disease outbreak in North Kivu and Ituri Provinces, Democratic Republic of the Congo – fourth update', ECDC: Stockholm, Available at: https://www.ecdc.europa.eu/en/publications-data/rapid-risk-assessment-ebola-virus-disease-outbreak-north-kivu-and-ituri-0 (accessed 31 July 2020).

187 European Centre for Disease Prevention and Control (2020), 'Risk assessment guidelines for infectious diseases transmitted on aircraft (RAGIDA)'. ECDC: Stockholm, Available at: https://www.ecdc.europa.eu/en/publications-data/risk-assessment-guidelines-infectious-diseases-transmitted-aircraft-ragida-middle (accessed 31 July 2020).

- Travellers who have stayed in a recently affected area should be made aware that if they develop symptoms compatible with COVID-19 within 14 days after arrival, they should self-isolate, contact health services and mention potential exposure to Covid-19. Secondary transmission to caregivers in the family and in healthcare facilities cannot be ruled out if no measures are taken for infection prevention and control.[188]

In order to minimise the time between onset of symptoms, isolation and diagnosis, people who return from COVID-19-affected areas should be informed about:

- the possibility of exposure to COVID-19 while in affected countries
- the clinical presentation of the disease and the need to seek immediate medical care if symptoms develop
- the need to immediately disclose their travel history when seeking medical care and to preferably do so before arriving at a healthcare facility

[188] European Centre for Disease Prevention and Control. (2019), 'Rapid risk assessment: Ebola virus disease outbreak in North Kivu and Ituri Provinces, Democratic Republic of the Congo – fourth update', ECDC: Stockholm, Available at: https://www.ecdc.europa.eu/en/publications-data/rapid-risk-assessment-ebola-virus-disease-outbreak-north-kivu-and-ituri-0 (accessed 31 July 2020).

- the need to indicate possible contact with sick individuals or wild animals while in the COVID-19-affected country; and
- how to contact public health authorities for support if infection is suspected.[189]

In addition, healthcare providers around the world should be informed of and sensitised to:

- the possibility of COVID-19 among returning travellers from affected areas
- the clinical presentation of the disease and need to enquire about travel history and contacts with family and friends visiting from COVID-19-affected countries
- the availability of protocols for the ascertainment of possible cases and procedures for referral to healthcare facilities; and
- the imperative need for strict implementation of barrier management, use of personal protective equipment and disinfection procedures in accordance with specific guidelines and WHO infection control

189 European Centre for Disease Prevention and Control. (2019), 'Rapid risk assessment: Ebola virus disease outbreak in North Kivu and Ituri Provinces, Democratic Republic of the Congo – fourth update', ECDC: Stockholm, Available at: https://www.ecdc.europa.eu/en/publications-data/rapid-risk-assessment-ebola-virus-disease-outbreak-north-kivu-and-ituri-0 (accessed 31 July 2020).

recommendations when providing care to COVID-19 cases.[190]

5.3 CLOSURE OF SCHOOLS AND RESTRICTIONS ON PUBLIC GATHERINGS AND PUBLIC TRANSPORT

Without evidence for effective treatments or a successful vaccine for COVID-19, physical distancing has been recommended to minimise transmission, and thus reduce risk for the most vulnerable in society. Physical distancing also therefore reduces pressure on public health and healthcare services, and allows time for the prevention and management of the disease.[191]

A recent study published by *The BMJ* established that physical distancing measures, such as closing schools, workplaces, and public transport, and restricting mass gatherings, are associated with a meaningful reduction in new COVID-19 cases. In this study, five commonly introduced physical distancing interventions in 149 countries were associated with on average a 13% reduction in the incidence of

---

[190] European Centre for Disease Prevention and Control. (2019), 'Rapid risk assessment: Ebola virus disease outbreak in North Kivu and Ituri Provinces, Democratic Republic of the Congo – fourth update', ECDC: Stockholm, Available at: https://www.ecdc.europa.eu/en/publications-data/rapid-risk-assessment-ebola-virus-disease-outbreak-north-kivu-and-ituri-0 (accessed 31 July 2020).

[191] ScienceDaily (2020), 'Earlier lockdown restrictions linked to greater reduction in new COVID-19 cases', Available at: https://www.sciencedaily.com/releases/2020/07/200715190744.htm (accessed 31 July 2020).

COVID-19. No additional benefit was found associated with closures of public transport when a combination of school closures, workplace closures, restrictions on mass gatherings, and restrictions of population movement (ie, lockdown) was in place. A greater reduction in incidence was observed when restriction on mass gatherings was included in the intervention combination, and when lockdown was implemented earlier along with school and workplace closures.[192]

In another study released on the 20th of May 2020 by disease modelers at Columbia University, it was said that 61.6% of deaths and 55% of infections nationwide could have been avoided if preventative measures in place on March 15 had been enacted a week earlier. That equates to about 35,927 deaths and 703,975 cases.[193] On March 15, 2020, the United States Centers for Disease Control and Prevention recommended that no gatherings with 50 people or more — including weddings, festivals, parades, concerts, sporting events or conferences — be held in the United States for the next eight weeks in one of the federal government's most sweeping efforts to slow the spread of the coronavirus.[194]

---

192 BMJ (2020), 'Physical distancing interventions and incidence of coronavirus disease 2019: natural experiment in 149 countries', Available at: https://www.bmj.com/content/370/bmj.m2743 (accessed 31 July 2020).

193 ABC News (2020), 'Study finds earlier coronavirus restrictions in US could have saved 36,000 lives. Trump calls it a 'political hit job.', Available at: https://abcnews.go.com/Politics/study-finds-earlier-coronavirus-restrictions-us-saved-36k/story?id=70808611 (accessed 31 July 2020).

194 The New York Times (2020), 'C.D.C. Gives New Guidelines, New York to Close Restaurants and Schools and Italian Deaths Rise', Available at:

5.4 FACEMASKS AND RESPIRATORS

Facemasks, or surgical masks, are primarily designed to protect the environment from particles expelled by the wearer. If fitted properly, and used and changed in accordance with manufacturers instructions, they provide a physical barrier to large droplets but will not provide full respiratory protection against smaller particles such as aerosols.[195] Available evidence suggests protection by masks in high transmission settings such as household and college settings, especially if used early, in some trials if combined with hand hygiene and if wearers are compliant.[196]

Respirators are more sophisticated than facemasks and are designed to protect the wearer from breathing in fine or very small airborne particles (i.e. aerosols), which might contain viruses and other microorganisms, in addition to larger droplets. They should be worn when performing procedures that have the potential to generate infectious aerosols; examples include intubation, extubation and related procedures. It is a legal

---

https://www.nytimes.com/2020/03/15/world/coronavirus-live.html (accessed 31 July 2020).

[195] UK Department of Health, Social Services and Public Safety (2011), 'UK Influenza Pandemic Preparedness Strategy', Available at: https://www.gov.uk/government/publications/review-of-the-evidence-base-underpinning-the-uk-influenza-pandemic-preparedness-strategy (accessed 29 July 2020).

[196] MacIntyre, C. R., & Chughtai, A. A. (2020). A rapid systematic review of the efficacy of face masks and respirators against coronaviruses and other respiratory transmissible viruses for the community, healthcare workers and sick patients. *International journal of nursing studies*, *108*, 103629. https://doi.org/10.1016/j.ijnurstu.2020.103629 (accessed 29 July 2020).

requirement that anyone who might be required to wear a respirator be fit-tested to ensure that an adequate seal can be achieved to provide the best level of protection and that training in use be provided. More than one make of respirator should be made available to help account for different face shapes among employees.[197]

5.5 CONTROLLING INFECTION IN HEALTH-CARE SETTINGS

Health-care workers should always take standard precautions when caring for patients, regardless of their presumed diagnosis. These include basic hand hygiene, respiratory hygiene, use of personal protective equipment (to block splashes or other contact with infected materials), safe injection practices and safe burial practices.[198]

5.5.1 CARE FOR PEOPLE WITH SUSPECTED OR CONFIRMED COVID-19

Health-care workers caring for patients with suspected or confirmed COVID-19 should apply extra infection control measures to prevent contact with the patient's blood and body

[197] UK Department of Health, Social Services and Public Safety (2011), 'UK Influenza Pandemic Preparedness Strategy', Available at: https://www.gov.uk/government/publications/review-of-the-evidence-base-underpinning-the-uk-influenza-pandemic-preparedness-strategy (accessed 29 July 2020).

[198] World Health Organization. Ebola virus disease [Internet]. Geneva: WHO; 2019 [cited 11 April 2019]. Available from: http://www.who.int/news-room/fact-sheets/detail/ebola-virus-disease (accessed 29 July 2020).

fluids and contaminated surfaces or materials such as clothing and bedding. When in close contact (within 1 metre) of patients with COVID-19, health-care workers should wear face protection (a face shield or a medical mask and goggles), a clean, non-sterile long-sleeved gown, and gloves (sterile gloves for some procedures).[199]

It is important to prioritize rapid diagnostic testing and confirmatory laboratory testing in pregnant women with suspected COVID-19, as they may require acute obstetric care and may pose a risk of COVID-19 transmission from pregnancy-related fluids and tissues. There may be considerable overlap in symptoms between early COVID-19 and pregnancy-related conditions in pregnant women. As such, evaluation of pregnant women by obstetric and COVID-19 trained healthcare providers is essential, and clinical management should be informed by risk of exposure to COVID-19, symptom history, and an obstetric evaluation. Pregnant women with suspected or confirmed COVID-19 should be evaluated and treated in designated spaces within COVID-19 treatment centers with measures to ensure privacy.[200]

---

[199] World Health Organization. Ebola virus disease [Internet]. Geneva: WHO; 2019 [cited 11 April 2019]. Available from: http://www.who.int/news-room/fact-sheets/detail/ebola-virus-disease (accessed 23 July 2020).

[200] World Health Organization (2020), 'Guidelines for the management of pregnant and breastfeeding women in the context of Ebola virus disease', Available at: https://www.who.int/publications/i/item/guidelines-for-the-management-of-pregnant-and-breastfeeding-women-in-the-context-of-ebola-virus-disease (accessed 23 July 2020).

Appropriate resources and personnel trained in obstetric and neonatal care should be available at COVID-19 treatment centers in order to avoid treatment delays or risks associated with transporting pregnant women. Specialist support can be provided by a mobile team who can come to the COVID-19 treatment centre or via telemedicine/telephone. The decision to manage obstetric complications in order to save the life of a pregnant woman with confirmed or suspected COVID-19 requires a case-by-case evaluation that takes into account maternal and not foetal indications, individual patient characteristics, as well as personnel and resource availability. Shared decision-making involving the patient, family members and healthcare workers is encouraged.[201]

To protect healthcare workers who are caring for patients with COVID-19, healthcare facilities must provide onsite management and oversight of adherence to safely using personal protective equipment (PPE), and implement administrative and environmental controls with continuous safety checks through direct observation of healthcare workers, including during the PPE donning and doffing steps.

201 World Health Organization (2020), 'Guidelines for the management of pregnant and breastfeeding women in the context of Ebola virus disease', Available at: https://www.who.int/publications/i/item/guidelines-for-the-management-of-pregnant-and-breastfeeding-women-in-the-context-of-ebola-virus-disease (accessed 23 July 2020).

Healthcare workers must follow the basic principles below to ensure that no infectious material reaches unprotected skin or mucous membranes while providing patient care.

Donning

- PPE must be donned correctly in proper order before entry into the patient care area; PPE should not be later modified while in the patient care area. The donning activities must be directly observed by a trained observer.

During Patient Care

- PPE must remain in place and be worn correctly for the duration of work in potentially contaminated areas. PPE should not be adjusted during patient care. In the event of a significant splash, the healthcare worker should immediately move to the doffing area to remove PPE. The one exception is that visibly contaminated outer gloves can be changed while in the patient room and patient care can continue. Contaminated outer gloves can be disposed of in the patient room with other COVID-19 associated waste.
- Healthcare workers should perform frequent disinfection of gloved hands using an **alcohol-based**

hand rub (ABHR), particularly after contact with body fluids.

- If during patient care any breach in PPE occurs (e.g., a tear develops in an outer glove, a needlestick occurs, a glove separates from the sleeve), the healthcare worker must move immediately to the doffing area to assess the exposure. The facility exposure management plan should be implemented; including correct supervised doffing and appropriate occupational health follow-up, if indicated by assessment. In the event of a potential exposure, bloodborne pathogen exposure procedures must be followed in accordance with the **Occupational Safety and Health Act of 1970 (OSHA) Bloodborne Pathogens Standard.**

DOFFING

- Removing used PPE is a high-risk process that requires a structured procedure, a trained observer, a doffing assistant in some situations, and a designated area for removal to ensure protection.
- PPE must be removed slowly and deliberately in the correct sequence to reduce the possibility of self-contamination or other exposure to COVID-19.

- A stepwise process should be developed and used during training and patient care.[202]

Double-gloving provides an easy way to remove gross contamination by changing an outer glove during patient care and when removing PPE. Beyond this, more layers of PPE may make it more difficult to perform patient care duties and put healthcare workers at greater risk for percutaneous injury (e.g., needlesticks), self-contamination during care or doffing, or other exposures to COVID-19. If healthcare facilities decide to add additional PPE or modify this PPE guidance, they must consider the risk/benefit of any modification and train healthcare workers on how to correctly don and doff for the modified procedure. Donning and doffing steps may need to be adapted on the basis of the specific PPE that is purchased by the hospital. If adaptations are made, facilities must select PPE that offers a similar or higher level of protection than what is recommended here, train healthcare workers in its use, and ensure they demonstrate competence in its use before caring for a patient with COVID-19.[203]

---

[202] United States Centers for Disease Control and Prevention, 'Guidance on Personal Protective Equipment (PPE) To Be Used By Healthcare Workers during Management of Patients with Confirmed Ebola or Persons under Investigation (PUIs) for Ebola who are Clinically Unstable or Have Bleeding, Vomiting, or Diarrhea in U.S. Hospitals, Including Procedures for Donning and Doffing PPE', Available at: https://www.cdc.gov/vhf/ebola/healthcare-us/ppe/guidance.html (accessed 25 July 2020).

[203] United States Centers for Disease Control and Prevention, 'Guidance on Personal Protective Equipment (PPE) To Be Used By Healthcare Workers during Management of Patients with Confirmed Ebola or Persons under Investigation (PUIs) for Ebola who are Clinically Unstable or Have Bleeding, Vomiting, or

Training ensures that healthcare workers are knowledgeable and proficient in donning and doffing PPE before caring for a patient with COVID-19. Comfort and proficiency when donning and doffing are only achieved by repeatedly practicing correct use of PPE. Healthcare workers should be required to demonstrate competency in using PPE, including donning and doffing while being observed by a trained observer, before working with patients with COVID-19. Training should be tailored to the intended audience and effectively transmit the required information. In addition, during practice, healthcare workers and their trainers should assess proficiency and comfort with performing required duties while wearing PPE. People unwilling or unable to fulfill these requirements should not care for a patient with COVID-19.[204]

The following elements are essential for PPE training:

- How to safely don, adjust, use, and doff the specific PPE that the healthcare worker will use;
- How to safely conduct routine clinical care;

Diarrhea in U.S. Hospitals, Including Procedures for Donning and Doffing PPE', Available at: https://www.cdc.gov/vhf/ebola/healthcare-us/ppe/guidance.html (accessed 25 July 2020).

204 United States Centers for Disease Control and Prevention, 'Guidance on Personal Protective Equipment (PPE) To Be Used By Healthcare Workers during Management of Patients with Confirmed Ebola or Persons under Investigation (PUIs) for Ebola who are Clinically Unstable or Have Bleeding, Vomiting, or Diarrhea in U.S. Hospitals, Including Procedures for Donning and Doffing PPE', Available at: https://www.cdc.gov/vhf/ebola/healthcare-us/ppe/guidance.html (accessed 25 July 2020).

- Limitations of the PPE (e.g., duration of use, degree of protection);
- What to do in the case of an equipment failure or detection of a breach in PPE;
- How to maintain PPE and appropriately dispose of it after use; and
- The possible physiologic strain associated with using PPE, and how to recognize and report early signs and symptoms, such as fatigue.
- Training must be interactive and should allow frontline healthcare workers to practice donning, adjusting, using, and doffing the specific PPE that the employee will use.
- Hospitals should ensure that the trained employees understand the content of the training and can correctly perform the required tasks.
- Hospitals should also ensure that employees can demonstrate how to properly don, use, and doff the same type/model PPE and respirators that they will use when caring for a patient.
- Regular refresher trainings are essential to maintaining these skills.[205]

---

205 United States Centers for Disease Control and Prevention, 'Guidance on Personal Protective Equipment (PPE) To Be Used By Healthcare Workers during Management of Patients with Confirmed Ebola or Persons under Investigation (PUIs) for Ebola who are Clinically Unstable or Have Bleeding, Vomiting, or Diarrhea in U.S. Hospitals, Including Procedures for Donning and Doffing PPE',

Laboratory workers are also at risk. Samples taken from humans and animals for investigation of COVID-19 infection should be handled by trained staff and processed in suitably equipped laboratories.[206]

5.5.2 CARE FOR PEOPLE WHO RECOVERED FROM COVID-19

COVID-19 survivors need comprehensive support for the medical and psychosocial challenges they face and also to minimize the risk of continued coronavirus transmission. To address these needs, a dedicated programme can be set up for care for people who recovered from COVID-19.[207]

After a Covid-19 survivor's condition stabilizes, but prior to discharge from the COVID-19 Treatment Unit (CTU), he or she should receive education and counselling regarding the possible sequelae and psycho-social challenges faced during convalescence. With permission, it is ideal to include consultation with the survivor's close family members, explaining in simple terms the common sequelae and what is known about how coronavirus can and cannot be transmitted during convalescence and what measures they can take to avoid

Available at: https://www.cdc.gov/vhf/ebola/healthcare-us/ppe/guidance.html (accessed 25 July 2020).

206 World Health Organization. Ebola virus disease [Internet]. Geneva: WHO; 2019 [cited 11 April 2019]. Available from: http://www.who.int/news-room/fact-sheets/detail/ebola-virus-disease (accessed 25 July 2020).

207 World Health Organization. Ebola virus disease [Internet]. Geneva: WHO; 2019 [cited 11 April 2019]. Available from: http://www.who.int/news-room/fact-sheets/detail/ebola-virus-disease (accessed 25 July 2020).

virus transmission. COVID-19 survivors should be given a follow-up appointment to see a care provider within 2-weeks after discharge and specific instructions about who to contact if they encounter health problems or have questions. Issues such as confidentiality, avoiding stigmatization, and cost of follow-up care should be addressed. In cases when significant mental health problems are noted before discharge or anticipated afterwards, it may be appropriate to refer patients directly to a mental health care provider.[208]

Following recovery from COVID-19, it is important to offer pregnant women comprehensive counselling on the risk of an adverse pregnancy outcomes and pregnancy management options. A woman may choose to proceed with an induced abortion, pregnancy induction, or expectant management. If an induced abortion is desired, the gestational age and the presence or absence of prior uterine surgeries should be taken into consideration. Guidance on medically induced abortions, including medication regimens, can be found in the WHO guideline "Medical management of abortion". Products of conception should be assumed to be potentially infectious until the COVID-19 testing has resulted. Because of this, it is necessary to use COVID-19-specific PPE (double gloves, face mask, gown or coverall and apron, head cover, eye protection

[208] World Health Organization (2020), 'Clinical care for survivors of Ebola virus disease: Interim Guidance', Available at: https://www.who.int/csr/resources/publications/ebola/guidance-survivors/en/ (accessed 23 July 2020).

(goggles or face shield) and boots, as well as standard precautions.[209]

At discharge, COVID-19 survivors should be provided with documents containing their unique patient ID, name, age, symptoms at presentation, and any convalescent symptoms at discharge, a brief record of their test results and treatment in the CTU, and their government or laboratory-issued COVID-19 Survivor's Certificate. This information will serve as a 'transfer of care' document for their outpatient management. Survivors should be instructed to bring these documents, as well as documents recording past vaccination, to all future clinic or hospital visits).[210]

5.6 CONTACT TRACING

Contact tracing is an integral component of the overall strategy for controlling an outbreak of an infectious disease. Contact tracing is defined as the identification and follow-up of persons who may have come into contact with an infected person.

---

209 World Health Organization (2020), 'Guidelines for the management of pregnant and breastfeeding women in the context of Ebola virus disease', Available at: https://www.who.int/publications/i/item/guidelines-for-the-management-of-pregnant-and-breastfeeding-women-in-the-context-of-ebola-virus-disease (accessed 23 July 2020).

210 World Health Organization (2020), 'Clinical care for survivors of Ebola virus disease: Interim Guidance', Available at: https://www.who.int/csr/resources/publications/ebola/guidance-survivors/en/ (accessed 23 July 2020).

In principle, contact tracing is broken down into three basic elements, namely, contact identification, contact listing and contact follow-up. The three elements of contact tracing are described below.

5.6.1 CONTACT IDENTIFICATION

Contact identification is an essential part of epidemiologic investigation for all cases meeting the standard/surveillance case definitions of infectious diseases like COVID-19. These cases are classified as suspected, probable or confirmed. Epidemiologic investigation is also conducted for all deaths, either in the community or in a health facility, that are attributable to infectious diseases. The process of verifying the cause of death is called verbal autopsy, which aims to establish the likely cause of death and identify chains of transmission. The tool for conducting an epidemiologic investigation is the case investigation form. The use of a comprehensive and standardized case investigation form is recommended. The epidemiologist/surveillance officer conducting the epidemiologic investigation should complete case investigation forms for all the infectious diseases cases and deaths meeting the standard/surveillance case definition.[211]

[211] World Health Organization (2014), 'Contact Tracing During an Outbreak of Ebola Virus Disease', Available at: https://www.who.int/csr/resources/publications/ebola/contact-tracing-during-outbreak-of-ebola.pdf (accessed 25 July 2020).

After completing the case investigation form, the epidemiologist/surveillance officer should systematically identify potential contacts. Contact identification therefore begins from a case. Identification of contacts is done by asking about the activities of the case (whether alive or dead) and the activities and roles of the people around the case (alive/dead) since onset of illness. Although some information can be obtained from the patient, much of the information will come from the people around the patient. In many instances, the patient will have died or have already been admitted to the isolation facility, with limited access. It is mandatory for the epidemiologist/surveillance officer to visit the home of the patient.[212]

5.6.2 CONTACT LISTING

All persons considered to have had significant exposure (falling in the categories described above) should be listed as contacts. Efforts should be made to physically identify every listed contact and inform them of their contact status, what it means, the actions that will follow, and the importance of receiving early care if they develop symptoms. The contact should also be

212 World Health Organization (2014), 'Contact Tracing During an Outbreak of Ebola Virus Disease', Available at: https://www.who.int/csr/resources/publications/ebola/contact-tracing-during-outbreak-of-ebola.pdf (accessed 25 July 2020).

provided with preventive information to reduce the risk of exposing people close to them.[213]

The process of informing contacts of their status should be done with tact and empathy, since being a contact can be associated with serious health outcomes. Avoid using alarming information, such as 'COVID-19 has no treatment' or 'COVID-19 has a very high case fatality rate'. Advise all contacts to:

(a). Remain at home as much as possible and restrict close contact with other people.

(b). Avoid crowded places, social gatherings, and the use of public transport.

(c). Report any suspicious signs and symptoms such as fever, headache, and weakness immediately (provide telephone numbers for the contact follow-up team, the supervisor or the COVID-19 hotline/call centre numbers). Explain that getting early and good clinical care improves health outcomes, and immediate evacuation from the home and isolation reduces the risk of infecting family members.

In addition, provide information on:

---

[213] European Centre for Disease Prevention and Control. Public health management of persons having had contact with Ebola virus disease cases in the EU – 7 November 2014. Stockholm: ECDC; 2014. Available from: http://ecdc.europa.eu/publications-data/public-health-management-persons-having-had-contact-ebola-virus-disease-cases-0 (accessed 25 July 2020).

(a). COVID-19 preventive measures through inter-personal communication and where applicable, provide materials like leaflets and brochures.

(b). Preventive measures to mitigate the risk of exposing family members and others if a contact develops symptoms.

(c). Guidance for home-based care at onset of illness while waiting for evacuation and isolation.

Contact identification and listing, including the process of informing contacts of their status, should be done by the epidemiologist or surveillance officer, not by the local surveillance staff/community health worker performing the daily follow-up. The local surveillance staff/community health worker should be introduced during the initial home visit as the person who will conduct home visits.[214]

5.6.3 CONTACT FOLLOW-UP

The epidemiologist/surveillance officer responsible for contact tracing should assemble a competent team comprising local surveillance and appropriate community members to follow up all the listed contacts. This could include surveillance

214 World Health Organization (2014), 'Contact Tracing During an Outbreak of Ebola Virus Disease', Available at: https://www.who.int/csr/resources/publications/ebola/contact-tracing-during-outbreak-of-ebola.pdf (accessed 25 July 2020).

staff/health workers from health facilities, community health workers, volunteers e.g. from the Red Cross and community leaders.

An efficient contact tracing system depends on a relationship of trust with the community, which in turn fosters optimum cooperation. Communities should have the confidence to cooperate with contact tracing teams and allow the referral of symptomatic contacts to designated isolation facilities. Involving appropriate community members (in particular local leaders) in contact tracing is critical in cultivating this good relationship, trust and confidence. The local surveillance and community volunteers should be involved as early as possible in the response. The local surveillance staff and community health workers should be closely supervised by trained epidemiologists/surveillance officers.[215]

Contact persons should immediately self-isolate and contact health services in the event of any symptom appearing within 2-14 days after exposure to the virus. If no symptoms appear within 14 days of last exposure the contact person is no longer considered to be at risk of developing COVID-19.[216]

---

[215] World Health Organization (2014), 'Contact Tracing During an Outbreak of Ebola Virus Disease', Available at: https://www.who.int/csr/resources/publications/ebola/contact-tracing-during-outbreak-of-ebola.pdf (accessed 25 July 2020).

[216] European Centre for Disease Prevention and Control. Public health management of persons having had contact with Ebola virus disease cases in the EU – 7 November 2014. Stockholm: ECDC; 2014. Available from: http://ecdc.europa.eu/publications-data/public-health-management-persons-having-had-contact-ebola-virus-disease-cases-0 (accessed 25 July 2020).

5.7 TREATMENT

Clinical management of COVID-19 should focus on supportive care of complications, such as Shortness of breath or difficulty breathing.

Recommended care includes volume repletion, maintenance of blood pressure (with vasopressors if needed), and maintenance of oxygenation, pain control, nutritional support, and treatment of secondary bacterial infections and pre-existing comorbidities. Large volumes of intravenous fluids are often required to correct dehydration due to diarrhea and vomiting. Some patients may develop profound third-spacing of fluids due to vascular leak. Some organizations suggest the addition of broad-spectrum antimicrobials, particularly in patients with evidence of septic shock. Infection prevention and control measures are a critical part of clinical management. Consider all bodily fluids and clinical specimens as potentially infectious.[217]

---

217 Centers for Disease Control and Prevention (2016), 'Ebola Virus Disease (EVD) Information for Clinicians in U.S. Healthcare Settings', Available at: https://www.cdc.gov/vhf/ebola/clinicians/evd/clinicians.html?CDC_AA_refVal=https%3A%2F%2Fwww.cdc.gov%2Fvhf%2Febola%2Fhealthcare-us%2Fpreparing%2Fclinicians.html (accessed 26 July 2020).

INDEX

REFERENCES ARE TO PARAGRAPH NUMBERS

A

AVIAN AND OTHER ZOONOTIC INFLUENZA
CASE DEFINITION, 1.1.6.
DIAGNOSIS, 1.1.6.
EPIDEMIOLOGY OF HUMAN INFECTIONS, 1.1.6.
PANDEMIC POTENTIAL, 1.1.6.
PREVENTION, 1.1.6.
SIGNS AND SYMPTOMS IN HUMANS, 1.1.6.
THE PATHOGEN, 1.1.6.
TRANSMISSION, 1.1.6.
TYPES OF INFLUENZA VIRUSES, 1.1.6.
WORLD HEALTH ORGANIZATION'S RESPONSE, 1.1.6.

C

CLOSURE OF SCHOOLS AND RESTRICTIONS ON PUBLIC GATHERINGS AND PUBLIC TRANSPORT, 5.3.

CONTACT TRACING
CONTACT FOLLOW-UP, 5.6.3.

CONTACT IDENTIFICATION, 5.6.1.
CONTACT LISTING, 5.6.2.

CONTROLLING INFECTION IN HEALTH-CARE SETTINGS
CARE FOR PEOPLE WHO RECOVERED FROM COVID-19, 5.5.2.
CARE FOR PEOPLE WITH SUSPECTED OR CONFIRMED COVID-19, 5.5.1.

COVID-19
CASE DEFINITION, 1.1.1.
DAILY LIFE AND GOING OUT, 1.1.1.
HISTORY, 1.1.1.
INCUBATION PERIOD, 1.1.1.
PREVENTING GETTING SICK, 1.1.1.
SYMPTOMS, 1.1.1.
TESTING, 1.1.1.
TRANSMISSION, 1.1.1.

E

EBOLA VIRUS DISEASE
CASE DEFINTION, 1.1.4.
DAILY LIFE AND GOING OUT, 1.1.4.
HISTORY, 1.1.4.
INCUBATION PERIOD, 1.1.4.
PEOPLE AT INCREASED RISK, 1.1.4.
PREVENTING GETTING SICK, 1.1.4.

SPECIES, 1.1.4.
SYMPTOMS, 1.1.4.
TESTING, 1.1.4.
TRANSMISSION, 1.1.4.
TRAVEL, 1.1.4.

EMERGING INFECTIOUS DISEASES
AVIAN AND OTHER ZOONOTIC INFLUENZA, 1.1.6.
COVID-19, 1.1.1.
EBOLA VIRUS DISEASE, 1.1.4.
HUMAN IMMUNODEFICIENCY VIRUS, 1.1.9.
MARBURG VIRUS DISEASE, 1.1.5.
MIDDLE EAST RESPIRATORY SYNDROME (MERS), 1.1.2.
PANDEMIC INFLUENZA, 1.1.8.
SEASONAL INFLUENZA, 1.1.7.
SEVERE ACUTE RESPIRATORY SYNDROME (SARS), 1.1.3.

F

FACEMASKS AND RESPIRATORS, 5.4.

FINANCIAL ACTION TASK FORCE'S APPROACH TO RISK ASSESSMENT
ANALYSIS, 3.2.2, 4.2.
EVALUATION, 3.2.3, 4.3.
IDENTIFICATION, 3.2.1, 4.1.

G

GLOBAL RISK ASSESSMENT
THE WORLD HEALTH ORGANIZATION, 2.0.

H

HIGHLY PATHOGENIC AVIAN INFLUENZA (HPAI) A(H5N1)
HISTORY, 1.1.6.
PREVENTING GETTING SICK, 1.1.6.
SYMPTOMS, 1.1.6.
TRANSMISSION, 1.1.6.
WHAT IS HIGHLY PATHOGENIC AVIAN INFLUENZA, 1.1.6.

HUMAN IMMUNODEFICIENCY VIRUS (HIV)
CASE DEFINTION, 1.1.9.
HISTORY, 1.1.9.
PREVENTING GETTING SICK, 1.1.9.
SYMPTOMS, 1.1.9.
TRANSMISSION, 1.1.9.

I

INTERNATIONAL HEALTH REGULATIONS (IHR) 2005
ARTICLE 1, 2.0.
ARTICLE 5, 2.0.

ARTICLE 6, 2.0.
ARTICLE 10, 2.0.
ARTICLE 11, 2.0.
ARTICLE 12, 2.0.
ARTICLE 15, 2.0.

INTERNATIONAL TRAVEL, BORDER RESTRICTIONS AND SCREENING, 5.2.

M

MARBURG VIRUS DISEASE
CASE DEFINTION, 1.1.5.
DAILY LIFE AND GOING OUT, 1.1.5.
HISTORY, 1.1.5.
INCUBATION PERIOD, 1.1.5.
PREVENTING GETTING SICK, 1.1.5.
SYMPTOMS, 1.1.5.
TESTING, 1.1.5.
TRANSMISSION, 1.1.5.
TREATMENT, 1.1.5.

MIDDLE EAST RESPIRATORY SYNDROME (MERS)
CASE DEFINITION, 1.1.2.
DIAGNOSIS, 1.1.2.
EPIDEMIOLOGY OF HUMAN INFECTIONS, 1.1.2.
PREVENTION, 1.1.2.
SIGNS AND SYMPTOMS IN HUMANS, 1.1.2.
THE PATHOGEN, 1.1.2.

TRANSMISSION, 1.1.2.
TREATMENT, 1.1.2.
WORLD HEALTH ORGANIZATION'S RESPONSE, 1.1.2.

N

NATIONAL RISK ASSESSMENT
NIGERIA, 2.3.
UNITED KINGDOM, 2.2.
UNITED STATES OF AMERICA, 2.1.

NIGERIA'S APPROACH TO COMBATING INFECTIOUS DISEASES
CONDUCT, COLLATE, SYNTHESIZE AND DISSEMINATE, 1.2.4.
CONTROL DISEASES OF PUBLIC HEALTH IMPORTANCE, 1.2.4.
COORDINATE SURVEILLANCE SYSTEMS, 1.2.4.
DETECT DISEASES OF PUBLIC HEALTH IMPORTANCE, 1.2.4.
DEVELOP AND MAINTAIN SPECIALSED LABORATORIES, 1.2.4.
PREVENT DISEASES OF PUBLIC HEALTH IMPORTANCE, 1.2.4.
SUPPORT STATES, 1.2.4.

P

PANDEMIC INFLUENZA
CASE DEFINITION, 1.1.8.
HISTORY, 1.1.8.
PLANNING PROCESS, 1.1.8.

PANDEMIC INFLUENZA PHASES
ALERT PHASE, 1.2.1.
INTERPANDEMIC PHASE, 1.2.1.
PANDEMIC PHASE, 1.2.1.
TRANSITION PHASE, 1.2.1.

R

REDUCING THE SPREAD OF DISEASE: INFECTION CONTROL & RESPIRATORY AND HAND HYGIENE
ADOPT THOROUGH RESPIRATORY AND HAND HYGIENE PRACTICES, 5.1.
AVOID CONSUMPTION OF BUSH MEAT AND CONTACT WITH WILD ANIMALS, 5.1.
AVOID CONTACT WITH SYMPTOMATIC PATIENTS, 5.1.
ENSURE SAFE SEXUAL PRACTICES, 5.1.
STAY AT HOME, 5.1.
WASH AND PEEL FRUIT AND VEGETABLES BEFORE CONSUMPTION, 5.1.

RISK

DEFINITION, 2.0, 3.0.
MEDICAL RISK ASSESSMENT, 1.2.1, 1.2.2, 1.2.3, 2.0.
MONEY LAUNDERING AND TERRORIST FINANCING RISK ASSESSMENT, 3.0, 3.1, 3.2.

RISK ANALYSIS, 2.0, 3.2.2, 4.2.

RISK ASSESSMENT

DEFINITION, 2.0.
DOSE-RESPONSE ASSESSMENT, 2.0.
EXPOSURE ASSESSMENT, 2.0.
GLOBAL RISK ASSESSMENT, 1.2.1, 1.2.2, 1.2.3, 2.0.
HAZARD IDENTIFICATION, 2.0.
INTERNATIONAL HEALTH REGULATIONS (IHR) 2005, 2.0.
NATIONAL RISK ASSESSMENT, 3.0, 3.1, 3.2, 3.2.1, 3.2.2, 3.2.3, 4.0, 4.1, 4.2, 4.3.

RISK CONTROL MEASURES

CLOSURE OF SCHOOLS AND RESTRICTIONS ON PUBLIC GATHERINGS AND PUBLIC TRANSPORT, 5.3.
CONTACT TRACING, 5.6.
CONTROLLING INFECTION IN HEALTH-CARE SETTINGS, 5.5.
FACEMASKS AND RESPIRATORS, 5.4.
INFECTION CONTROL & RESPIRATORY AND HAND HYGIENE, 5.1.
INTERNATIONAL TRAVEL, BORDER RESTRICTIONS AND SCREENING, 5.2.
TREATMENT, 5.7.

RISK EVALUATION, 2.0, 3.2.3, 4.3.

RISK IDENTIFICATION, 2.0, 3.2.1, 4.1.

RISK MANAGEMENT CYCLE
IDENTIFICATION OF POTENTIAL CONTROL MEASURES, 2.0.
MONITORING AND EVALUATION, 2.0.
RISK ASSESSMENT, 2.0.

S

SEASONAL INFLUENZA
CASE DEFINITION, 1.1.7.
THE PATHOGEN, 1.1.7.
SIGNS AND SYMPTOMS IN HUMANS, 1.1.7.
EPIDEMIOLOGY OF HUMAN INFECTIONS, 1.1.7.
TRANSMISSION, 1.1.7.
DIAGNOSIS, 1.1.7.
TREATMENT, 1.1.7.
PREVENTION, 1.1.7.
WORLD HEALTH ORGANIZATION'S RESPONSE, 1.1.7.
TYPES OF SEASONAL INFLUENZA VIRUSES, 1.1.7.

SEVERE ACUTE RESPIRATORY SYNDROME (SARS)
CASE DEFINITION, 1.1.3.
HISTORY, 1.1.3.
INCUBATION PERIOD, 1.1.3.
PREVENTING GETTING SICK, 1.1.3.

SYMPTOMS, 1.1.3.
TRANSMISSION, 1.1.3.

T

THE GLOBAL APPROACH TO COMBATING INFECTIOUS DISEASES
THE WORLD HEALTH ORGANIZATION, 1.2.1.
UNITED KINGDOM'S DEPARTMENT OF HEALTH, SOCIAL SERVICES AND PUBLIC SAFETY, 1.2.3.
UNITED STATES CENTERS FOR DISEASE CONTROL AND PREVENTION, 1.2.2.

TREATMENT, 1.1.1, 1.1.2, 1.1.3, 1.1.4, 1.1.5, 1.1.6, 1.1.7, 1.1.8, 1.1.9, 5.7.

U

UNITED KINGDOM'S APPROACH TO COMBATING INFECTIOUS DISEASES
ASSESSMENT, 1.2.3.
DETECTION, 1.2.3
ESCALATION, 1.2.3.
RECOVERY, 1.2.3.
TREATMENT, 1.2.3.

UNITED STATES' APPROACH TO COMBATING INFECTIOUS DISEASES

PHASE 1: ASSESS CURRENT STATE, 1.2.2.

PHASE 2: DETERMINE STRATEGIES AND ACTIVITIES, 1.2.2.

PHASE 3: DEVELOP PLANS, 1.2.2.

W

WORLD HEALTH ORGANIZATION'S APPROACH TO COMBATING INFECTIOUS DISEASES

GLOBAL PANDEMIC PHASES, 1.2.1.

EHI ERIC ESOIMEME'S PUBLICATIONS

BOOKS

- Esoimeme E, E. (2020), 'Application programming interfaces and Artificial intelligence-enabled systems', Sanction Scanner (eds), Expected Changes in AML After Covid-19, 1st Edition, Sanction Scanner, Turkey, 13 – 14, https://sanctionscanner.com/Static/Ebooks/Expected-Changes-in-AML-after-COVID-19.pdf
- Esoimeme, E.E. (2019),'The Risk-Based Approach to Combating Modern Slavery', DSC Publications Ltd, Available on Amazon: https://www.amazon.co.uk/Risk-Based-Approach-Combating-Modern-Slavery/dp/9782787914/ref=sr_1_fkmr0_1?keywords=ehi+esoimeme&qid=1569793632&s=gateway&sr=8-1-fkmr0
- Esoimeme, E.E. (2019), 'Balancing Anti-Money Laundering/Counter-Terrorist Financing Requirements and Financial Inclusion: The Case of

Telecommunications Companies', DSC Publications Ltd, Available on Amazon: https://www.amazon.co.uk/Balancing-Anti-Money-Laundering-Counter-Terrorist-Requirements/dp/9782787892/ref=sr_1_1?keywords=esoimeme&qid=1559731958&s=gateway&sr=8-1

- Esoimeme, E.E. (2018), 'Deterring and Detecting Money Laundering and Terrorist Financing: A Comparative Analysis of Anti–Money Laundering and Counterterrorism Financing Strategies', DSC Publications Ltd, Available on Amazon: https://www.amazon.co.uk/Deterring-Detecting-Laundering-Terrorist-Financing/dp/9782787795/ref=sr_1_1?ie=UTF8&qid=1520869556&sr=8-1&keywords=ehi+esoimeme
- Onwudiwe, C.C. and Esoimeme, E.E. (2016), 'Banker-Customer Relationship: A Practical Legal Guide', Bank Customers Association of Nigeria.
- Esoimeme, E.E. (2015), 'The Risk-Based Approach to Combating Money Laundering and Terrorist Financing', Eric Press; Available on Amazon: https://www.amazon.co.uk/Risk-Based-Combating-Laundering-Terrorist-Financing/dp/9789486030/ref=sr_1_2?ie=UTF8&qid=1437508453&sr=8-2&keywords=ehi+eric+esoimeme

- Esoimeme, E.E. (2014), 'A Comparative Study of the Money Laundering Laws/Regulations in Nigeria, the United States and the United Kingdom', Eric Press; Available on Amazon: https://www.amazon.co.uk/dp/9782787906/ref=sr_1_5?keywords=ehi+esoimeme&qid=1570888055&sr=8-5

ARTICLES

- Esoimeme, E.E. (2020), "Identifying and reducing the money laundering risks posed by individuals who have been unknowingly recruited as money mules", *Journal of Money Laundering Control*, Vol. ahead-of-print No. ahead-of-print. https://doi.org/10.1108/JMLC-05-2020-0053
- Esoimeme, E.E. (2020), "Leveraging Anti-Money Laundering Policies and Procedures to Combat Illicit Trafficking in Narcotic Drugs" Available at SSRN: https://ssrn.com/abstract=3613697 or http://dx.doi.org/10.2139/ssrn.3613697
- Esoimeme, E.E. (2020), "Balancing anti-money laundering measures and financial inclusion: The example of the United Kingdom and Nigeria", *Journal of Money Laundering Control*, Vol. 23 No. 1, pp. 64-76. https://doi.org/10.1108/JMLC-04-2018-0031

- Esoimeme, E.E. (2020), "Institutionalising the war against corruption: new approaches to assets tracing and recovery", *Journal of Financial Crime*, Vol. ahead-of-print No. ahead-of-print. https://doi.org/10.1108/JFC-12-2018-0125
- Esoimeme, E.E. (2020), "Using the risk-based approach to curb modern slavery in the supply chain: The Anglo American and Marks and Spencer example", *Journal of Financial Crime*, Vol. ahead-of-print No. ahead-of-print. https://doi.org/10.1108/JFC-05-2019-0056
- Esoimeme, E.E. (2020), "Using anti-money laundering measures to curb pension fraud in Nigeria", *Journal of Financial Crime*, Vol. ahead-of-print No. ahead-of-print. https://doi.org/10.1108/JFC-12-2018-0126
- Esoimeme, E.E. (2019), "Using the lie detector test to curb corruption in the Nigerian Police Force", *Journal of Financial Crime*, Vol. 26 No. 3, pp. 874-880. https://doi.org/10.1108/JFC-06-2018-0058
- Esoimeme E.E. (2019), 'The Abacha Case: How AML Procedures Should Have Flagged $267m Earlier', KYC360 (the global financial crime and compliance knowledge hub powered by RiskScreen), https://www.riskscreen.com/kyc360/article/the-abacha-case-how-aml-procedures-should-have-flagged-267m-earlier/?

- Esoimeme E.E. (2019), 'Enhancing Financial Inclusion: Telecoms and AML in Nigeria', KYC360 (the global financial crime and compliance knowledge hub powered by RiskScreen), https://www.riskscreen.com/kyc360/research-papers/enhancing-financial-inclusion-telecoms-and-aml-in-nigeria/
- Esoimeme, E.E. (2019), "A critical analysis of the anti-corruption policy of the federal executive council of Nigeria", *Journal of Money Laundering Control*, Vol. 22 No. 2, pp. 176-187. https://doi.org/10.1108/JMLC-06-2017-0021
- Esoimeme, E.E. (2018), "A comparative analysis of the prepaid card laws/regulations in Nigeria, the UK, the USA and India", *Journal of Money Laundering Control*, Vol. 21 No. 4, pp. 481-493. https://doi.org/10.1108/JMLC-03-2017-0010
- Esoimeme, E.E. (2018), 'Banking: Curbing employee fraud and corruption with an effective KYE program', KYC360 (the global financial crime and compliance knowledge hub powered by RiskScreen), https://www.riskscreen.com/kyc360/article/banking-curbing-employee-fraud-and-corruption-with-an-effective-kye-program/
- Esoimeme E.E. (2018), 'Fighting Corruption? It's Worth Considering a Preventive Approach to Asset

Recovery', KYC360 (the global financial crime and compliance knowledge hub powered by RiskScreen), https://kyc360.com/article/fighting-corruption-its-worth-considering-a-preventive-approach-to-asset-recovery/

- Esoimeme, E.E. (2018), "A critical analysis of the anti-corruption policy of the national judicial council of Nigeria", *Journal of Money Laundering Control*, Vol. 21 No. 3, pp. 253-263. https://doi.org/10.1108/JMLC-01-2017-0001
- Esoimeme, E.E. (2018), "The money laundering risks and vulnerabilities associated with MMM Nigeria", *Journal of Money Laundering Control*, Vol. 21 No. 1, pp. 112-119. https://doi.org/10.1108/JMLC-01-2017-0002
- Esoimeme, E. (2017), "A critical analysis of the effects of the Central Bank of Nigeria foreign exchange policy on financial inclusion, anti-money laundering measures and fundamental rights", *Journal of Money Laundering Control*, Vol. 20 No. 4, pp. 417-427. https://doi.org/10.1108/JMLC-05-2016-0020
- Esoimeme, E.E. (2017), "The Nigerian Money Laundering (Prevention and Prohibition) Bill, 2016: a critical appraisal", *Journal of Money Laundering Control*, Vol. 20 No. 1, pp. 79-88. https://doi.org/10.1108/JMLC-07-2016-0025
- Esoimeme, E.E. (2016), 'Wealth Management, Tax Evasion and Money Laundering: The Panama Papers

Case Study', Law Digest Issue 11 Autumn 2016. Available at Law Digest: https://issuu.com/nglawdigest/docs/law_digest_issue_11_autumn_2016

- Esoimeme, E.E. (2016), 'Balancing Anti-Money Laundering/Counter-Terrorist Financing Requirements and Financial Inclusion for Migrants: A Case Study of Germany', Available at SSRN: https://ssrn.com/abstract=2710097
- Esoimeme, E.E. (2015), 'A Critical Analysis of the Bank Verification Number Project Introduced by the Central Bank of Nigeria', Available at SSRN: https://ssrn.com/abstract=2544934 or http://dx.doi.org/10.2139/ssrn.2544934
- Esoimeme, E.E. (2015), 'A Comparative Study of the Money Laundering Laws/Regulations in Nigeria, the United States and the United Kingdom: Reporting Requirements', Professionals Center for Business Research Volume 2 – June 2015 (06). Available at SSRN: https://ssrn.com/abstract=2441086
- Esoimeme, E.E. (2015), 'The Death Penalty: An Effective Anti-Corruption Mechanism?', Available at SSRN: https://ssrn.com/abstract=2621268
- Esoimeme, E.E. (2015), 'A Critical Analysis of the Anti-Money Laundering Measures Adopted by BitGold Inc', Available at SSRN: https://ssrn.com/abstract=2604721 or http://dx.doi.org/10.2139/ssrn.2604721

- Esoimeme, E.E. (2014), 'Has the Concept of Plea Bargaining Been Abused in Nigeria's Criminal Justice System?', The Legal Aid Journal Volume 1. Available at SSRN: https://ssrn.com/abstract=2462307
- Esoimeme, E.E. (2014), 'A Comparative Study of the Money Laundering Laws/Regulations in Nigeria, the United States and the United Kingdom: Cash Couriers', The PUNCH, VOL 38 NO. 20,733, 20,739 PAGE 25, 29. Available at SSRN: https://ssrn.com/abstract=2476587
- Esoimeme, E.E. (2013), 'A Critical Analysis of the Effect of the Double Criminality Test on the Investigation Team and the Prosecution's Case', Available at SSRN: https://ssrn.com/abstract=2514719
- Esoimeme, E.E. (2013), 'A Critical Analysis of the Effect of the Double Criminality Test on Nominated Officers and Money Laundering Reporting Officers (MLRO) in the Regulated Sector', Available at SSRN: https://ssrn.com/abstract=2462952
- Esoimeme, E.E. (2013), 'The Importance of Why Firms Dealing with PEPs Must Adopt a Risk-Based Approach to Their Compliance Programmes', Available at SSRN: https://ssrn.com/abstract=2430972

EHI ERIC ESOIMEME HAS EDITED THE FOLLOWING PUBLICATIONS:

- Deji Sasegbon Esq., SAN (2020), 'Sasegbon's Judicial Dictionary of Nigerian Law (the first comprehensive judicial dictionary in Nigeria in 7 Volumes)', *DSC Publications.*
- Deji Sasegbon Esq., SAN (2015), 'Sasegbon on Election Petitions', *DSC Publications.*, Volume 3 Part III and 12 other volumes.

EHI ERIC ESOIMEME HAS ALSO PEER REVIEWED THE FOLLOWING PUBLICATIONS:

- Ross, I. (2015), 'Exposing Fraud: Skills, Process and Practicalities', Wiley Corporate F&A. Available on Amazon: https://www.amazon.co.uk/Exposing-Fraud-Process-Practicalities-Corporate-ebook/dp/B01CJK4Z8Q/ref=sr_1_fkmr0_2?ie=UTF8&qid=1493990138&sr=8-2-fkmr0&keywords=ian+ross+on+fraud
- Nwachukwu, E. (2015), 'Academic Excellence in 21 Days', Partridge Africa. Available on Amazon: https://www.amazon.co.uk/Academic-Excellence-Days-Eric-Nwachukwu/dp/1482826224/ref=sr_1_1?ie=UTF8&qid=1493990393&sr=8-1&keywords=eric+nwachukwu

www.ingramcontent.com/pod-product-compliance
Lightning Source LLC
Chambersburg PA
CBHW071447230926
51846CB00001B/371
* 9 7 8 9 7 8 2 7 8 7 9 2 7 *